Viva and Structured Oral Examinations

in
Intensive
Care
Medicine

Jeyasankar Jeyanathan, Chris Johns

tfm Publishing Limited, Castle Hill Barns, Harley, Shrewsbury, SY5 6LX, UK
Tel: +44 (0)1952 510061; Fax: +44 (0)1952 510192
E-mail: info@tfmpublishing.com
Web site: www.tfmpublishing.com

Editing, design & typesetting: Nikki Bramhill BSc Hons Dip Law
Cover photos: © iStockphoto LP — www.istockphoto.com
From left to right: monitoring the patient's vitals is a priority (PeopleImages); seriously ill patients in intensive care unit (sudok1); monitoring of mechanically ventilated patient (sudok1); all for the treatment of the patient (sudok1)

First edition:	© 2018	
Paperback	ISBN: 978-1-910079-59-1	
E-book editions:	2018	
Epub	ISBN: 978-1-910079-60-7	
Mobi	ISBN: 978-1-910079-61-4	
Web pdf	ISBN: 978-1-910079-62-1	

Printed by Cambrian Printers, Llanbadarn Road, Aberystwyth, Ceredigion, SY23 3TN, UK
Tel: +44 (0)1970 627111; Web site: www.cambrian-printers.co.uk

Contents

Preface

The British Fellowship of the Faculty of Intensive Care Medicine (FFICM) is a relatively new examination, with elements similar to the Australia and New Zealand Fellowship of the College of Intensive Care Medicine (FCICM) exam, the European Diploma of Intensive Care Medicine (EDIC) exam and other UK Royal College examinations. It is a rigorous assessment consisting of a multiple-choice question (MCQ) examination, objective structured oral examination (OSCE) and a structured oral examination (SOE), as a standard set, aimed at "a doctor in training who is familiar with the syllabus and has done the necessary bookwork. They would clinically be at the level of a registrar who would be able to formulate a plan of care for a critically ill patient with appropriate consultant backup"[1]. When we successfully completed the FFICM in 2014-15, there were very few dedicated resources available to turn to for 'bookwork', particularly for the SOE. This book is the culmination of our many hours of study, compiling material and question-spotting, that we thought may be of use to others in a similar position.

It is worth noting that none of us are involved in the setting or assessment of any examinations in ICM, but these vivas are a realistic representation of those we faced. Indeed, many of the topics covered have come up and will no doubt come up again. This book is targeted at the viva elements of the FFICM, European Diploma in Intensive Care Medicine (EDIC), the FCICM, and the ICM components of the final FRCA and other international examinations in intensive care.

1. The Faculty of Intensive Care Medicine. *Critical Eye* 2015; Issue 8, Summer 2015: 21. https://www.ficm.ac.uk/sites/default/files/critical_eye_8_-_summer_2015_final_website2. pdf.

Viva and Structured Oral Examinations in Intensive Care Medicine provides a comprehensive overview of 42 topics, with representative questions and model answers based on current evidence, that will stand you in good stead when facing these verbal assessments. Furthermore, this book will provide valuable rehearsal in the skill of presenting a suitably succinct and accurate answer for areas in the curriculum of both familiarity and rarity. We hope you find it a valuable resource and we wish you all the very best in your endeavours.

Jeyasankar Jeyanathan
Chris Johnson
James Haslam

Contributors

Nicholas A Barrett
BSc (Med) (Hons) MBBS (Hons) FANZCA FCICM AFICM
Consultant in Anaesthetics and Intensive Care Medicine
Guy's and St Thomas' NHS Foundation Trust, London, UK

James D Haslam
BSc (Hons) DPMSA MBBS AKC FRCA FFICM
Consultant in Anaesthetics and Intensive Care Medicine
Salisbury NHS Foundation Trust, Wiltshire, UK

Nicholas Jonathan Hoare
BSc (Hons) MBBS FHEA PGCert (Clinical Education) FRCA
Specialty Registrar in Anaesthetics and Intensive Care Medicine
King's College Hospitals NHS Foundation Trust, London Deanery, UK

Jeyasankar Jeyanathan
BMedSci (Hons) MBBS DMCC PGCert (Med Sim) FRCA FFICM
Consultant in Anaesthetics and Intensive Care Medicine
Defence Medical Services, UK
Defence Lecturer, National Institute of Academic Anaesthesia
Academic Department of Military Anaesthesia and Critical Care

Christopher Johnson
MBBS FRCA FFICM DMCC DipIMC(RCSEd)
Consultant in Anaesthetics and Intensive Care Medicine
The Royal Victoria Infirmary, Newcastle upon Tyne, UK

Sqn Ldr Alexandra Nelson
MBBS
Specialty Registrar in Anaesthetics and Intensive Care Medicine
Defence Medical Services, UK

Abbreviations

AAA	Abdominal aortic aneurysm
ABG	Arterial blood gas
AChR	Acetylcholine receptors
ADH	Antidiuretic hormone
ADRT	Advance decision to refuse treatment
ALS	Advanced life support
ALT	Alanine aminotransferase
ANP	Atrial natriuretic peptide
APACHE	Acute Physiology and Chronic Health Evaluation
APP	Abdominal perfusion pressure
ARDS	Acute respiratory distress syndrome
AST	Aspartate aminotransferase
ATC	Automatic tube compensation
AV	Atrioventricular
BIVAD	Biventricular assist device
BMI	Body mass index
BP	Blood pressure
BPS	Behavioural Pain Scale
BTS	British Thoracic Society
CAM-ICU	Confusion Assessment Method for the Intensive Care Unit
CCPOT	Critical Care Pain Observation Tool
CK	Creatine kinase
CKD	Chronic kidney disease
Cl^-	Chloride
cmH_2O	Centimetres of water
CNS	Central nervous system
CO_2	Carbon dioxide
COPD	Chronic obstructive pulmonary disease
CPAP	Continuous positive airway pressure
CPP	Cerebral perfusion pressure
CPR	Cardiopulmonary resuscitation
CRE	Carbapenem-resistant enterobacteriaceae

CRP	C-reactive protein
CSF	Cerebrospinal fluid
CSWS	Cerebral salt wasting syndrome
CT	Computed tomography
CTPA	Computed tomography pulmonary angiography
CVA	Cerebrovascular accident
CVC	Central venous catheter
CVP	Central venous pressure
CXR	Chest X-ray
DAD	Diffuse alveolar damage
DAT	Direct antiglobulin test
DBD	Donation after brainstem death
DCD	Donation after circulatory death
DI	Diabetes insipidus
DIC	Disseminated intravascular coagulation
DKA	Diabetic ketoacidosis
DNA	Deoxyribonucleic acid
DoLS	Deprivation of Liberty Safeguards
ECF	Extracellular fluid
ECG	Electrocardiography
ECMO	Extracorporeal membrane oxygenation
EEG	Electroencephalography
ERCP	Endoscopic retrograde cholangiopancreatography
ESBL	Extended-spectrum beta-lactamase
ETT	Endotracheal tube
FBC	Full blood count
FEV_1	Forced expiratory volume in 1 second
FFP	Fresh frozen plasma
FiO_2	Fractional concentration of inspired oxygen
FRC	Functional residual capacity
FRIII	Fixed rate intravenous insulin infusion
GCS	Glasgow Coma Scale
GEDI	Global End-Diastolic Volume Index
GFR	Glomerular filtration rate
GMC	General Medical Council
Hb	Haemoglobin
HELLP	Haemolysis, elevated liver enzymes and low platelets
HHS	Hyperosmolar hyperglycaemic state

HIT	Heparin-induced thrombocytopenia
HIV	Human immunodeficiency virus
HUS	Haemolytic uraemic syndrome
IABP	Intra-aortic balloon pump
IAH	Intra-abdominal hypertension
IAP	Intra-abdominal pressure
ICNARC	Intensive Care National Audit and Research Centre
ICP	Intracranial pressure
ICU	Intensive care unit
IMCA	Independent mental capacity advocate
INR	International Normalised Ratio
ISS	Injury Severity Score
ITBI	Intrathoracic Blood Volume Index
IV	Intravenous
IVC	Intravenous catheter
IVIg	Intravenous immunoglobulin
kPa	Kilo Pascals
LAST	Local anaesthetic systemic toxicity
LDH	Lactate dehydrogenase
LRP	Lipoprotein receptor-related protein
LV	Left ventricle
LVAD	Left ventricular assist device
MAHA	Microangiopathic haemolytic anaemia
MAOI	Monoamine oxidase inhibitor
MAP	Mean arterial pressure
MCA	Mental Capacity Act
MELD	Model of End-stage Liver Disease
MG	Myasthenia gravis
MHC	Major histocompatibility complex
MIP	Maximum inspiratory pressure
mmHg	Millimetres of mercury
MODS	Multiple Organ Dysfunction Score
MRI	Magnetic resonance imaging
MRSA	Methicillin-resistant *Staphylococcus aureus*
MuSK	Muscle-specific tyrosine kinase
Na^+	Sodium
NAPQI	N-acetyl-p-benzoquinone
NEWS	National Early Warning Score

NICE	National Institute for Health and Care Excellence
NIF	Negative inspiratory force
NIV	Non-invasive ventilation
NMB	Neuromuscular blocking drugs
NMJ	Neuromuscular junction
NMS	Neuroleptic malignant syndrome
NPSA	National Patient Safety Agency
PALS	Patient Advocacy and Liaison Service
PaO_2	Partial pressure of oxygen in arterial blood
PCR	Polymerase chain reaction
PEA	Pulseless electrical activity
PEEP	Positive end-expiratory pressure
PEFR	Peak expiratory flow rate
P-POSSUM	Portsmouth Physiological and Operative Severity Score for the enUmeration of Mortality
PPE	Personal protective equipment
PRC	Packed red blood cells
PVL	Panton-Valentine leukocidin
QDS	*Quater die sumendum* — 4 times a day
RAS	Renin angiotensin system
RASS	Richmond Agitation Sedation Scale
RCT	Randomised controlled trial
RDOS	Respiratory Distress Observation Scale
RNA	Ribonucleic acid
ROSC	Return of spontaneous circulation
ROTEM®	Rotational thromboelastometry
RSBI	Rapid Shallow Breathing Index
RV	Right ventricle
RVAD	Right ventricular assist device
SAPS	Simplified Acute Physiology Score
SAS	Sedation-Agitation Score
SBT	Spontaneous breathing trial
SC	Subcutaneous
SIADH	Syndrome of inappropriate antidiuretic hormone secretion
SIMV	Sychronised intermittent mandatory ventilation
SIRS	Systemic inflammatory response syndrome
SJS	Stevens-Johnson syndrome
SLE	Systemic lupus erythematosus

SOFA	Sequential Organ Failure Assessment
SSC	Surviving Sepsis Campaign
SSRI	Selective serotonin reuptake inhibitor
SVV	Stroke volume variation
TACO	Transfusion-associated circulatory overload
TBSA	Total body surface area
TEG®	Thromboelastography
TEN	Toxic epidermal necrolysis
TIPSS	Transjugular intrahepatic portosystemic shunt
TISS	Therapeutic Intervention Scoring System
TIVA	Total intravenous anaesthesia
TMA	Thrombotic microangiopathy
TRALI	Transfusion-related acute lung injury
TRC	Tube resistance compensation
TTP	Thrombotic thrombocytopenic purpura
TURP	Transurethral resection of the prostate
U&Es	Urea and electrolytes
VAC	Vacuum-assisted closure
VAD	Ventricular assist device
VAP	Ventilator-acquired pneumonia
VILI	Ventilator-induced lung injury
V/Q	Ventilation/perfusion
VRE	Vancomycin-resistant enterococci
VTEC	Verotoxin-producing *Escherichia coli*
WBC	White blood cell

Dedication

To our teachers and colleagues, thank you. To our patients and their loved ones, thank you for allowing us to be a part of your lives.

To my mother and father and beautiful family; the love in my life, inspiration, drive and best friend, and the two angel boys in our lives. Thank you.

J Jeyanathan

To Clare who puts up with me, guides me and loves me. Thank you for all that you do.

Chris

To my wife Emily, for persevering with me through many exams. Thank you for encouraging me to pursue my passion.

J Haslam

SET 1

1) What is the mortality following cardiac arrest?

The mortality rates vary significantly depending upon the cause of the cardiac arrest, the age of the patient and the setting in which they arrest. The survival to hospital discharge for all-cause out-of-hospital cardiac arrest in England is 8.6%. The classic consensus was that the out-of-hospital cardiac arrest patients who had early bystander CPR, who were in a shockable rhythm and who were defibrillated early had a better outcome than in-hospital slowly deteriorating patients who were usually in a non-shockable rhythm and had no immediate reversible causes but generalised physiological decline.

2) What is the post-cardiac arrest syndrome?

The post-cardiac arrest syndrome is characterised by the following triad:

- Myocardial dysfunction — also called myocardial 'stunning', affecting the heart globally. Early echocardiography will therefore show very poor function, but this generally improves. If the stunning is so severe that there is a low cardiac output despite adequate filling and appropriate peripheral vascular resistance, then the stunned heart may respond well to positive inotropy. Early echocardiography should therefore be avoided unless there is suspicion of valve rupture or a left ventricular aneurysm as a result of the initial insult.

- Reperfusion syndrome — reperfusion of ischaemic tissue releases cytokines and hypoxic metabolites into the circulation. This causes vasoplegia and impaired oxygen utilisation in all tissues. It can also cause hypotension which may be responsive to vasopressor therapy and adequate intravascular filling.
- Hypoxic brain injury — hypoxaemia results in the primary insult of brain cell apoptosis, plus the secondary insult of impaired cerebral autoregulation and subsequent cerebral oedema. This should be managed with the same neuroprotective measures as for head injury, with careful attention to oxygenation and appropriate ventilation, cerebral perfusion pressure maintenance, strict sodium, glucose and seizure control.

3) What are the management priorities post-cardiac arrest?

General management

- The airway should be protected appropriate to the patient's Glasgow Coma Scale (GCS) score, which may include intubation and mechanical ventilation. Care should be taken to ensure adequate oxygenation and ventilation to a normal $PaCO_2$ for cerebral protection. Similarly, hyperoxia may be harmful in the post-arrest period.
- Sedation — whilst there are no data to support this, it is standard practice to sedate patients to allow physiological settling and to 'rest' the brain. Patients who have had a degree of hypoxic ischaemic cerebral insult may become very agitated in the immediate post-arrest period.
- Cerebral perfusion pressure needs to be maintained — the hypoxic ischaemic time may have affected cerebral autoregulation, with cerebral perfusion dependent upon mean arterial pressure which should therefore be maintained through a combination of fluid resuscitation, inotropes and vasopressors, as required.

Specific management

- The cause of cardiac arrest should be identified and if possible reversed — specifically, patients who have suffered a primary cardiac event should have their coronary arteries catheterised and revascularised.
- Hyperthermia should be avoided (see below).
- Maintenance of normoglycaemia using insulin and dextrose infusions as appropriate — there is a good correlation between poor glucose control post-cardiac arrest and poor neurological outcome.
- Control of seizures if present — seizures increase the cerebral metabolic rate significantly and therefore may further damage an already injured brain. There is a lack of evidence, but seizure prophylaxis post-cardiac arrest should be considered in patients who have had a significant hypoxic-ischaemic cerebral insult.

4) Should we be cooling patients post-cardiac arrest?

There has been conflicting evidence in the recent past regarding cooling post-cardiac arrest:

- Evidence for: two studies from Europe and Australia showed that patients cooled post-arrest had no survival benefit but had a more favourable neurological outcome. Criticism of these trials included the large exclusion rate and the high incidence of hyperthermia in the control group — essentially, they compared hypothermia to hyperthermia.
- Evidence against: a 2013 trial compared cooling to 33°C with targeted temperature management of 36°C and showed no difference in mortality or neurological outcome.

Therefore, the current consensus opinion is that the avoidance of hyperthermia is on a par with therapeutic hypothermia in terms of neurological outcome, and avoids the potential complications associated with cooling patients.

5) How can we prognosticate patients post-cardiac arrest on intensive care?

Predicting outcome following return of spontaneous circulation (ROSC) after a cardiac arrest is difficult to achieve.

Factors associated with a poor outcome include:

- Unwitnessed arrest with no bystander CPR.
- Pulseless electrical activity (PEA)/asystole as the initial rhythm.
- Basic life support (CPR only) for greater than 10 minutes prior to advanced life support — specifically the time to defibrillation.
- Advanced life support for greater than 20 minutes prior to ROSC.

Whilst these may be associated with a poor outcome generally, they are not specific enough for individual patient prognostication.

More specific predictors of poor neurological outcome at 72 hours include:

- Absence of pupillary or corneal reflexes.
- Motor score of 2 or less on the GCS.
- Myoclonic status epilepticus — this should not be confused with post-hypoxic myoclonus (Lance-Adams syndrome) which features intention myoclonus and is associated with recovery of consciousness and a much better prognosis.
- Raised neurone-specific enolase (>33μg/L).
- Absence of the N2O spike on somatosensory-evoked potentials bilaterally.
- Burst suppression or epileptiform discharges indicative of hypoxic ischaemic encephalopathy on EEG.

It is important to note that some intensive care units may not have routine access to the latter investigation modalities.

Summary of Key Points

- Mortality post-cardiac arrest depends upon the specific situation, patient, rhythm and time to treatment.
- Post-cardiac arrest syndrome consists of a triad of myocardial dysfunction, reperfusion injury and hypoxic brain injury.
- Post-arrest management is aimed at preventing secondary brain injury (primary being the hypoxic ischaemic insult).
- The avoidance of hyperthermia is superior to therapeutic hypothermia.
- Prognostication post-cardiac arrest is complex and cannot be reliably perfomed until >72 hours.

References

1. UK Resuscitation Council Consensus Paper on Out-of-Hospital Cardiac Arrest in England. Available from: https://www.resus.org.uk/publications/consensus-paper-on-out-of-hospital-cardiac-arrest-in-england/.

2. Laurent I, Monchi M, Chiche JD, *et al*. Reversible myocardial dysfunction in survivors of out-of-hospital cardiac arrest. *J Am Coll Cardiol* 2002; 40: 2110.

3. Nishizawa H, Kudoh I. Cerebral autoregulation is impaired in patients resuscitated after cardiac arrest. *Acta Anaesthesiol Scand* 1996; 40: 1149.

4. Bernard SA, Gray TW, Buist MD, *et al*. Treatment of comatose survivors of out-of-hospital cardiac arrest with induced hypothermia. *N Engl J Med* 2002; 346(8): 557-63.

5. The Hypothermia after Cardiac Arrest (HACA) Study Group. Mild therapeutic hypothermia to improve the neurologic outcome after cardiac arrest. *N Engl J Med* 2002; 346(8): 549-56.

6. Nielsen N, Wetterslev J, Cronberg T, *et al*. Targeted temperature management at 33°C versus 36°C after cardiac arrest. *N Engl J Med* 2013; 369: 2197.

7.   Wijdicks EF, Hijdra A, Young GB, *et al*. Practice parameter: prediction of outcome in comatose survivors after cardiopulmonary resuscitation (an evidence-based review): report of the Quality Standards Subcommittee of the American Academy of Neurology. *Neurology* 2006; 67: 203-10.

ARDS and prone ventilation

1) What is ARDS?

The classification of acute respiratory distress syndrome (ARDS) is shown below in ● Table 1.1.

Table 1.1. Berlin definition of ARDS.

Timing	Within 1 week of known clinical insult or new worsening respiratory symptoms.	
Chest imaging	Bilateral opacities — not fully explained by effusions, lobar/lung collapse or nodules.	
Origin of oedema	Respiratory failure not fully explained by cardiac failure or fluid overload. Need an objective assessment (e.g. echocardiography) to exclude hydrostatic oedema if no risk factors are present.	
ARDS severity	**PaO_2/FiO_2 (kPa, mmHg) with PEEP ≥5**	**Mortality (in study cohort)**
Mild	≤39.9kPa 200-300mmHg	27%
Moderate	≤26.6kPa 100-200mmHg	32%
Severe	≤13.3kPa <100mmHg	45%

2) What are the risk factors for the development of ARDS?

- Infective — sepsis, pneumonia.
- Trauma — fat embolism, drowning, burns, fractures, particularly multiple fractures and long bone fractures, with or without pulmonary contusion.
- Allergic/immunological/inflammatory — pancreatitis, reperfusion injury after cardiopulmonary bypass, aspiration, massive transfusion, transfusion-related acute lung injury (TRALI).
- Iatrogenic — drug overdose.
- Congenital — genetic susceptibility is under investigation.

For any illness a higher severity score (e.g. Acute Physiology and Chronic Health Evaluation — APACHE) increases the risk of ARDS.

3) What is the pathophysiology of ARDS?

ARDS is a combination of diffuse alveolar damage (DAD) and lung capillary endothelial injury; both cause increased permeability of the alveolar-capillary barrier.

Diffuse alveolar damage

Normal alveolar function depends upon Type 1 and Type 2 pneumocytes also called alveolar cells. Type 1 cells comprise 90% of alveolar epithelium. Type 1 cell damage increases fluid moving into the alveoli and decreases clearance. Type 2 pneumocytes have several functions including surfactant production, ion transport and differentiation into Type 1 to repair damage. Injury to Type 2 pneumocytes can reduce the production of surfactant, which contributes to atelectasis and worsening gas exchange.

Lung capillary endothelial injury

Meanwhile, damage to the microvascular endothelium results in increased permeability which allows movement of protein-rich exudate into the alveolar space.

The main site of injury depends on the disease process, for example, vascular endothelium in sepsis or alveolar epithelium in aspiration.

During ventilation, the less damaged and therefore more compliant alveoli may become over-distended, resulting in barotrauma. Damaged alveoli may be further injured from the forces exerted by the cycle of collapse and expansion though positive pressure ventilation.

4) What investigations would you do in someone you suspected had ARDS?

Bedside

- Echocardiography — useful for excluding cardiac causes of pulmonary oedema as per the diagnostic criteria.
- Lung ultrasound can demonstrate pleural line abnormalities, non-homogenous B-lines consistent with oedema, reduced lung sliding and consolidation which may aid the initial diagnosis.

Laboratory

- PaO_2/FiO_2 ratio <300mmHg is required for an ARDS diagnosis.
- U&Es — the patient is at risk of pre-renal failure if utilising a 'dry' fluid balance to reduce oedema.
- Coagulation screen — endothelial damage causes coagulation derangement.

Radiological

- The diagnosis of ARDS requires bilateral opacities on either chest CT or X-ray.
- CXR showing bilateral patchy infiltrates consistent with pulmonary oedema. Serial films are likely to be taken as the syndrome progresses.

- CT of the thorax can be used if there is diagnostic uncertainty but is not required.

Special

- Bronchoscopy — can evaluate the possibility of infection or haemorrhage and take material for microscopy, culture and staining which will assist with accurate antimicrobial therapy for infective causes.

5) A) What are the management principles in ARDS?

General

- Treat the underlying cause.
- Aim for an SpO_2 of >88% — ARDS usually requires mechanical ventilation.

Pharmacological

- No treatment has been shown to deliver an evidence-based benefit.

Ventilatory strategy

- Protective lung ventilation strategy — low-volume tidal ventilation of 6ml/kg (ideal body weight), plateau pressure of <30cm H_2O.
- Aim to maintain acceptable gas exchange while minimising adverse effects of mechanical ventilation.
- Positive end-expiratory pressure (PEEP) — to maintain alveolar recruitment. This should be tailored and titrated, for example, through a PEEP ladder system.
- Mean airway pressure — promote recruitment and predict adverse haemodynamics.
- Plateau pressure — predicts alveolar distension.

Management of refractory hypoxia

- High PEEP improves oxygenation but not mortality in moderate to severe ARDS.
- Prone positioning.
- Neuromuscular blockade for 48 hours in patients with moderate to severe ARDS has been demonstrated by randomised controlled trials to improve mortality and increase ventilator and organ failure-free days without any difference in ICU-acquired paresis.
- Conservative fluid therapy in patients with a lack of evidence of tissue hypoperfusion led to a reduced ICU stay with altering mortality.
- Oscillatory ventilation has been evaluated in six randomised controlled trials and has not been shown to improve survival.
- Extracorporeal membrane oxygenation (ECMO) — referral to an ECMO centre improves mortality and is cost effective.

B) What is the evidence for prone ventilation in ARDS?

The Proning Severe ARDS (PROSEVA) trial found a marked mortality benefit in ARDS patients with PF ratios >150 (i.e severe ARDS); NNT 6. Prone positioning has previously been shown to reduce over-distension and improve recruitment compared to supine ventilation. Prone positioning can improve patient outcome; however, the centres used in the PROSEVA trial were experienced with this technique. Awareness of the possible risks are key to avoiding adverse events.

C) What are the possible complications of prone ventilation and how can they be mitigated against?

- Once in the prone position, airway complications can be more difficult to recognise and rectify; for example, endotracheal tube displacement.

- Other complications include:
  - pressure sores, for example, genitalia, knee and face including the eye;
  - increased intracranial pressure;
  - increased intra-abdominal pressure.
- Well prepared and adequate staffing, correct patient choice, preparation to support pressure areas and the abdomen, and taking particular care with any drains or lines can help prevent adverse events.

D) Describe the postulated mechanisms by which prone positioning aids oxygen exchange in ARDS.

- Supine ventilation causes a reduced functional residual capacity (FRC).
- Prone ventilation:
  - improves V/Q matching as blood flow is increased to the dependent lung tissue;
  - reduced atelectasis;
  - less abdominal distension leads to a greater FRC;
  - heart rests on the sternum reducing compression of the left lung.

The effect of ventilation-related stress is more evenly distributed, reducing over-distension of alveoli and improving recruitment.

Summary of Key Points

- ARDS is hypoxaemia, bilateral opacities on chest imaging and pulmonary oedema not caused by cardiac failure or fluid overload.

- Mortality remains high at 40% and patients who are at risk should be identified. Lung-protective ventilation can reduce the exposure of patients to unnecessary risk factors.
- Patients with severe ARDS who are on or approaching maximal conventional therapy should be discussed with an ECMO centre.

References

1. Gattinoni L, Carlesso E. Prone positioning improves survival in severe ARDS: a pathophysiologic review and individual patient meta-analysis. *Minerva Anestesiologica* 2010; 76(6): 448-54.

2. Acute Respiratory Distress Syndrome (ARDS) definitions. LITFL - Life in the Fast Lane Medical Blog, 2014. Available from: https://lifeinthefastlane.com/ccc/acute-respiratory-distress-syndrome-ards-definitions/.

3. Acute respiratory distress syndrome. *JAMA* 2012; 307(23): 2526-33.

4. Mackay A, Al-Haddad M. Acute lung injury and acute respiratory distress syndrome. *Contin Educ Anaesth Crit Care Pain* 2009; 9(5): 152-6.

5. Guérin C, Reignier J, Richard J, *et al*. Prone positioning in severe acute respiratory distress syndrome. *N Engl J Med* 2013; 368(23): 2159-68.

6. Galiatsou E, Kostanti E, Svarna E, *et al*. Prone position augments recruitment and prevents alveolar overinflation in acute lung injury. *Am J Resp Crit Care Med* 2006; 174(2): 187-97.

7. Briel M, Meade M, Mercat A, *et al*. Higher vs. lower positive end-expiratory pressure in patients with acute lung injury and acute respiratory distress syndrome. *JAMA* 2010; 303(9): 865.

8. Gu X, Wu G, Yao Y, *et al*. Is high-frequency oscillatory ventilation more effective and safer than conventional protective ventilation in adult acute respiratory distress syndrome patients? A meta-analysis of randomized controlled trials. *Crit Care* 2014; 18(3): R111.

9. Noah M, Peek G, Finney S, *et al*. Referral to an extracorporeal membrane oxygenation center and mortality among patients with severe 2009 influenza A (H1N1). *JAMA* 2011; 306(15): 1659.

10. Danbury C, Gould T. Guidelines for the provision of intensive care services. Faculty of Intensive Care Medicine, 2016. Available from: https://www.ficm.ac.uk/sites/default/files/gpics_ed.1.1_-_2016_-_final_with_covers.pdf.

Haemolytic uraemic syndrome and thrombotic thrombocytopenic purpura

1) What is haemolytic uraemic syndrome (HUS)?

- HUS is one of the thrombotic microangiopathies and predominantly a disease of childhood characterised by a triad of:
  - haemolytic anaemia;
  - thrombocytopenia;
  - acute renal failure.
- It is a medical emergency with a mortality rate of up to 10%.
- HUS can be divided into two forms:
  - typical (D+ HUS) — accounting for 90% of cases in children, often with a 2-3-day prodrome of gastroenteritis associated with bloody diarrhoea, with strains of verotoxin-producing *Escherichia coli* (VTEC) being the likely causative organism;
  - atypical (D- HUS) — largely due to one of several genetic mutations that cause chronic, uncontrolled and excessive complement activation.
- Both forms cause:
  - endothelial cell damage;
  - leukocyte and platelet activation;
  - systemic thrombotic microangiopathy (thrombocytopenia, haemolysis);
  - thrombotic events;
  - widespread inflammation;
  - multi-organ failure;
  - ultimately, death.

2) List some laboratory markers of haemolysis.

- Anaemia.
- Elevated LDH.
- Reticulocytosis.

15

- Raised unconjugated bilirubin.
- Decreased haptoglobin.
- Negative direct Coombs or antiglobin tests.
- Blood film reveals fragmented erythrocytes (shistocytes).

3) A) How might you diagnose an *E. coli* infection?

- Stool culture.
- Some strains require specific molecular techniques, so document any suspicion of HUS on the request form.

B) What other pathogens may be causative?

- *Shigella*.
- *Streptococcus pneumoniae*.
- *Campylobacter*.
- Viruses.

4) A) How does HUS differ from thrombotic thrombocytopenic purpura (TTP)?

- TTP is another of the thrombotic microangiopathies that may present with the same triad as HUS, although renal involvement in TTP is rare.
- TTP tends to affect adults and additionally often presents with cardiac involvement (elevated troponin) and neurological disturbance including:
    - headache;
    - confusion;
    - hemiparesis;
    - seizures;
    - altered conscious level.

- However, diagnosis of TTP only requires the presence of microangiopathic haemolysis and thrombocytopenia with no alternative explanation.
- TTP, like HUS, can be congenital or acquired. Precipitating causes of TTP include:
  - cancer;
  - bone marrow transplantation;
  - HIV infection;
  - pregnancy;
  - medications.
- Haemolysis in TTP is the result of platelet microthrombi shearing red cells, and schistocytes on blood film is an essential finding.
- TTP is caused by a deficiency of, or antibodies against, serum metalloprotease ADAMTS13.
- ADAMTS13 is responsible for cleaving large von Willebrand factor multimers and deficiency allows unusually large multimers to remain in the circulation, resulting in multiple platelet aggregates.
- Undetectable or very low plasma levels of ADAMTS13 enzymatic activity (<10%) establish a diagnosis of TTP unequivocally.

B) What laboratory findings can help differentiate HUS and TTP from disseminated intravascular coagulation (DIC)?

- In DIC there will be:
  - an abnormal coagulation screen;
  - low fibrinogen;
  - high D-dimers.

5) A) Outline the treatment priorities for HUS.

- Treatment is largely supportive, including:
  - fluid and electrolyte imbalance correction;
  - nutritional support;

- haemodynamic support;
- renal replacement therapy.
- The use of antibiotics to treat *E. coli* diarrhoea is generally not advised as it may lead to progression to HUS.
- Platelet transfusion may worsen the outcome.

B) Discuss the role of plasma exchange.

- Plasma exchange has a proven role in TTP treatment and should be commenced urgently in all suspected cases.
- Plasma exchange in HUS is more controversial, although it may have a role in those cases with severe CNS involvement.
- The theory is that it removes the triggers leading to thrombotic microangiopathy including antibodies to ADAMTS13.

Summary of Key Points

- HUS and TTP, thrombotic microangiopathies, both present with haemolytic anaemia and thrombocytopenia. HUS tends to affect children and also features acute renal failure. TTP tends to affect adults and also features cardiac and CNS involvement.
- Both HUS and TTP can be congenital or acquired, with VTEC the likely precipitating organism in typical HUS.
- ADAMTS13 levels below 10% is pathognomonic for TTP.
- Treatment for both conditions is generally supportive, although plasma exchange is indicated in all cases of suspected TTP.

References

1. Dodd A, Dudley J, Twigg S. Plasma exchange in haemolytic-uremic syndrome secondary to *E. Coli* 026. *J Intensive Care Soc* 2013; 14(4): 343-5.
2. Thachil J. Thrombotic thrombocytopenic purpura. *J Intensive Care Soc* 2011; 12(3): 215-20.

Tricyclic antidepressant overdose

1) What are tricyclic antidepressants and what is their mechanism of action?

- Tricyclic antidepressants are based on phenothiazine and have a three-ringed structure.
- They inhibit neuronal reuptake of noradrenaline and serotonin in the central nervous system.
- Increased neurotransmitter levels at the synaptic cleft are thought to result in antidepressant effects.
- They are also used for the treatment of chronic pain, anxiety and migraine.
- Overdose is a common presentation to acute hospitals.

2) What are the features of tricyclic antidepressant overdose?

Features of tricyclic antidepressant overdose are a result of antagonism of muscarinic acetylcholine receptors, histamine H1 receptors, alpha-1 adrenoceptors and fast sodium channels on the cardiac myocyte. Severe toxicity develops with ingestion of more than 10mg/kg.

Clinical features

- Mild toxicity manifests as a syndrome of sympathomimetic excess with pupillary dilatation, dry mouth and skin, tachycardia, urinary retention and agitation.
- Severe toxicity results in decreased consciousness, seizures, hypotension, hypothermia, arrhythmia and respiratory depression.

Biochemical features

- Metabolic acidosis is a feature of severe toxicity.

Electrocardiographic features

- QTC interval prolongation.
- Arrhythmias.
- Widened QRS complex.
- R/S ratio greater than 0.7 in aVR.

3) How would you manage tricyclic antidepressant overdose?

Management should follow an 'airway, breathing, circulation, disability and exposure' pattern, with simultaneous resuscitation and assessment:

- High-flow oxygen should initially be given to all patients with a suspected severe overdose, and then titrated to achieve a PaO_2 of greater than 10kPa.
- Intubation is usually required if the initial GCS is less than 8.
- Activated charcoal may reduce absorption from the gastrointestinal tract if given within 1 hour of ingestion.
- ECG changes should be treated with intravenous sodium bicarbonate with a target plasma pH of 7.5.
- Benzodiazepines should be used to control seizures. Phenytoin should be avoided due to action on cardiac sodium channels.
- Adrenaline is favoured over noradrenaline for the treatment of fluid-refractory hypotension.
- Glucagon may be of benefit in the treatment of arrhythmia.
- Intravenous lipid emulsion has successfully been used for the treatment of cardiac arrest secondary to tricyclic antidepressant overdose.

4)   What are the clinical features of serotonin syndrome?

Serotonin syndrome affects about 10% of those presenting with overdose of selective serotonin reuptake inhibitors. Neuroleptic malignant syndrome is a differential diagnosis but presents with hyporeflexia instead of the hyperexciteability state of serotonin syndrome.

Clinical features

- Ocular clonus.
- Myoclonus.
- Hyperreflexia.
- Hyperthermia.
- Hypertension.
- Agitation.
- Arrhythmia.
- Autonomic instability.

5)   How would you manage serotonin syndrome?

- Hyperthermia can be life-threatening and should be controlled aggressively with cold intravenous fluids, cold lavage, ice packs and the use of fans.
- Endotracheal intubation and muscle relaxation with a non-depolarising neuromuscular blocking drug are indicated for temperatures greater than 41°C.
- Short-acting intravenous beta-blockers such as esmolol should be used to treat severe hypertension and tachycardia, once the fluid deficit from sweating has been corrected.
- Cyproheptadine is the specific treatment for serotonin syndrome, and is used if the above measures fail to control symptoms.

Summary of Key Points

- Tricyclic antidepressants work by increasing noradrenaline and serotonin concentrations at the synaptic cleft.
- Tricyclic antidepressant overdose is potentially life-threatening with an initial syndrome of sympathetic excess followed by decreased consciousness, coma and cardiac toxicity.
- Sodium bicarbonate should be used in severe toxicity to achieve a pH of 7.50.
- Serotonin syndrome may result in life-threatening hyperthermia, muscle rigidity and arrhythmia.
- Serotonin syndrome should be treated with measures to reduce body temperature, short-acting beta-blockade, and cyproheptadine in severe cases.

References

1. Body R, Bartram T, Azam F, Mackway-Jones K. Guidelines in Emergency Medicine Network (GEMNet): guideline for the management of tricyclic antidepressant overdose. *Emerg Med J* 2011; 28(4): 347-68.
2. Nordstrom K, Vilke GM, Wilson MP. Psychiatric emergencies for clinicians: emergency department management of serotonin syndrome. *J Emerg Med* 2016; 50(1): 89-91.

Statistics, evidence and research

1) What do you understand by the terms 'level of evidence' and 'grade of recommendation'?

These terms pertain to the strength of evidence based upon the quality and number of studies from which it was derived. The strength of this evidence then gives various grades of recommendation to translate academic work into clinical practice as described below.

Levels of evidence

- Level 1A — systematic review or meta-analysis of randomised controlled trials (RCT) (with homogeneity).
- Level 1B — individual RCT (with narrow confidence intervals).
- Level 1C — 'all or nothing' RCT (e.g. when all patients died before a treatment was available and now some survive on it or when some died before the treatment became available and now all survive).
- Level 2A — systematic review of cohort studies (with homogeneity).
- Level 2B — individual cohort study or low quality RCT.
- Level 2C — retrospective outcome data.
- Level 3A — systematic review of case-control studies (with homogeneity).
- Level 3B — individual case-control study.
- Level 4 — case series or poor quality cohort or case-control study.
- Level 5 — expert opinion.

Grade of recommendation

- Grade A — based on level 1 evidence.
- Grade B — based on consistent level 2 or 3 studies, or extrapolated from level 1 evidence.
- Grade C — based on level 4 studies, or extrapolated from level 2 or 3 studies.

- Grade D — based on level 5 evidence, or inconsistent/inconclusive studies from any level.

2) What is a meta-analysis?

A meta-analysis is a statistical technique used to combine several studies which are addressing similar research questions in order to increase the statistical power of the evidence. The output of the meta-analysis itself needs to be analysed — if poor quality studies are combined, then a meta-analysis may not add any value and give false elevation of poor evidence. Similarly, if very heterogeneous study populations are included then this can lead to bias.

3) What are the phases of clinical trials?

The introduction of a new medicine or intervention starts with pre-clinical, laboratory-based studies (Phase 0) — usually *in vitro* in nature and these are then followed by animal studies. Once these have been completed and human trials are sanctioned, there are several phases leading up to, and then following, the granting of a product licence.

Human trials are then commenced with the drug tested in the following phases:

- Phase 1 — 20-100 healthy volunteers — with the aim of determining pharmacokinetic and pharmacodynamic effects in humans.
- Phase 2 — 100-300 patients — further pharmacokinetic and dynamic data, at different doses and frequencies of administration.
- Phase 3 — 300-3000 patients — RCTs, comparing treatment against other or established therapies and/or placebo. Data are obtained on therapeutic effects and side effects.

After phase 3 trials, a product licence may be granted, but data are still collected in phase 4:

- Phase 4 — surveillance data during routine drug use in a larger population, so rare side effects may be discovered during this phase.

4) What types of data are you aware of?

Data can be divided into several types. Firstly, it is important to differentiate between population and sample data:

- Population data contains all the data from an entire study population.
- Sample data attempts to represent the entire population using a smaller group taken from it.

The advantage of sample data is that the smaller sample is easier to collect and analyse — this advantage needs to be weighed against the risk that the sample may not represent the entire population and therefore incorrect conclusions may be drawn.

Different types of data that can be collected are described below:

- Qualitative data (also called categorical) is split into:
  - nominal — data with no significant numerical order, e.g. blood group;
  - ordinal — data with an order of magnitude, e.g. severity scoring such as grade of subarachnoid haemorrhage.
- Quantitative data (also called numerical) is split into:
  - continuous — data which can take any value, e.g. weight;
  - discrete — data with finite values — such as numbers of ICU beds;
  - ratio — data with zero as its baseline, e.g. Kelvin temperature;
  - interval — data which includes zero on its scale but it isn't the base value, e.g. Centigrade temperature.

5) What is the difference between sensitivity and specificity?

- Sensitivity refers to the ability of a test to correctly predict a positive outcome where one exists. It can be calculated by dividing the number of results correctly identified as positive by the total number that were actually positive.
- Specificity refers to the ability of a test to correctly predict a negative outcome where one exists. It can be calculated by dividing the number of results correctly identified as negative by the total number that were actually negative.

6) What do you understand by the term 'p-value'?

The p-value, or probability value, is the likelihood of any outcome observed being a result of chance alone. Conventionally, statistical significance is taken at a p-value of 0.05, i.e. there is a 5% chance that the outcome observed is due to chance and a 95% chance that it is due to the intervention being investigated.

7) What are confidence intervals?

Confidence intervals are a range around a sample mean that will contain the true population mean at the stated value. For example, 95% confidence intervals are 95% confident that the true population mean will be within the range around the sample mean.

8) What is the 'Student's t-test' used for?

The Student's t-test is used for continuous parametric (normally distributed) data and can be used on paired or unpaired data to compare sample means. It is calculated by dividing the difference between the sample mean by the estimated standard error of the difference. This value is then referred to a table to determine if it represents statistical significance at the level of probability required.

27

9) How does 'analysis of variance' (ANOVA) differ from the 'Student's t-test'?

Unlike the Student's t-test which compares two sample means, the analysis of variance (ANOVA) test allows the comparison of three or more means; therefore, this is useful if more than two groups are being compared. A similar result could be achieved by undertaking multiple t-tests between each group, but by using ANOVA there is a smaller risk of detecting a false positive (Type I error).

Summary of Key Points

- The strength of guidelines and recommendations are based upon the quality of the evidence available. The better the evidence the stronger the recommendation.
- Meta-analysis can be a powerful tool to increase statistical evidence of a treatment effect. They still need to be critically appraised to ensure that they are adding value to a subject.
- Clinical trials are highly regulated, and most do not make it through to the latter stages. Data are still collected even after a drug or intervention is being used in routine clinical practice.
- There are many statistical tests, each used for a specific set of data to determine how accurately it represents the population being studied.

References

1. Pocock SJ. *Clinical trials: A Practical Approach.* Wiley, 1982.
2. Campbell MJ, Machin D. In: *Medical Statistics: A Common-sense Approach*, 2nd Ed. Wiley, 1993: 2.
3. Swinscow TDV. *Statistics at Square One*, 9th ed. BMJ Publishing Group, 1997.

Necrotising fasciitis

1) What is necrotising fasciitis and can you provide a classification?

- Necrotising fasciitis is a life-threatening soft-tissue infection primarily involving the superficial fascia.
- Although it is often clinically confused with cellulitis, this is a dangerous condition to misdiagnose, as necrotising fasciitis occurs suddenly and rapidly progresses in a destructive manner.
- Unfortunately, the disease process is often diagnosed quite late in its clinical course.
- It has a high mortality rate — approximately 30%.
- It can affect the lower or upper extremities, the abdominal wall or the perineum and genital area when it is often referred to as Fournier's gangrene.

Classification

Classification is based on microbiological findings and the responsible pathogens.

Type I or polymicrobial
- Accounts for most cases, approximately 70%.
- Obligate and facultative anaerobes.
- Anaerobic bacteria that proliferate in a hypoxic environment and produce gas. These accumulate in soft tissue spaces.
- Affects the trunk and perineum.
- Fournier's gangrene is typically a polymicrobial infection with aerobes and anaerobes, such as coliforms, *Klebsiella*, *Streptococci*, *Staphylococci*, *Clostridia*, *Bacteroides*, and *Corynebacteria*.

Type II or monomicrobial
- Beta-haemolytic *Streptococcus* A.

- *Streptococcus pyogenes* and *Staphylococcus aureus*.
- Affects the limbs.

Type III

- *Clostridium* species and Gram-negative bacteria.
- *Vibrio spp.*
- Affects the limbs, trunk and perineum.

Type IV

- Fungal, *Candida spp.*
- Limbs, trunk and perineum.
- Rapidly progressive, especially if immunocompromised.

A second classification can be based purely on monomicrobial or polymicrobial necrotising fasciitis.

Monomicrobial pathogens

- *Streptococci* (especially *Streptococcus pyogenes* — Group A).
- *Clostridium perfringens* (gas gangrene) and other clostridial species.
- *Staphylococcus aureus*.
- *Vibrio vulnificus*.
- *Aeromonas hydrophila*.

Polymicrobial pathogens

- Mixed aerobe-anaerobe bacterial flora (*E.coli, Bacteroides fragilis, Streptococci* and *Staphylococci*).

2) What patient groups and risk factors are associated with necrotising fasciitis?

The high mortality and morbidity with necrotising fasciitis is associated with late diagnosis and chronic disease or immunosuppressive states.

Patient groups and risk factors

Poor immune state

- Drug-related immunosuppressive states, for example, chronic steroid use, chemotherapy.
- Diabetes mellitus.
- Malignancy.
- Intravenous drug use.
- Excess alcohol use.
- Peripheral vascular disease.
- Chronic renal failure.
- Liver disease.
- Odontogenic infection.
- Chicken pox.

Trauma

- Surgery, for example, urgent or semi-elective surgery for wound debridement or intra-abdominal pathology.
- Penetrating trauma — large or small — for example, an animal bite.

3) Briefly outline the pathophysiology of necrotising fasciitis.

The hypodermis or the superficial fascia is where the bacteria, toxins and the interaction with enzymes and host factors occur. This synergistic interaction causes the infective destruction of the fat and fascia allowing the process to extend rapidly. Compounding this further is the bacterial interruption of the microcirculation in the hypodermis, thus causing ischaemia and, hence, further cellular death and necrosis. Anaerobic bacteria thrive in these conditions, producing gas as they proliferate, hence the crepitus.

4)   A) How can you diagnose this clinically?

The clinical status of the patient determines the most important set of diagnostics:

- Early non-specific changes include: erythema, swelling and tenderness.
- Advanced stages will feature: skin ischaemia, blisters and bullae.
- Disseminated and fulminant disease will portray a critically ill patient with signs and symptoms of severe septic shock and multiple organ dysfunction.

Infection of the lower extremities is the most common site of necrotising fasciitis at approximately 60%, followed by the abdomen 30% and the perineum 10%.

B) What investigations would you order and what might you see for someone with suspected necrotising fasciitis?

- A definitive diagnosis is attained by exploratory surgery at the infected sites.
- X-rays, computed tomography (CT), magnetic resonance imaging (MRI) and ultrasonography can be helpful, but no investigation should delay definitive surgical intervention in a suspected case of necrotising fasciitis.

Bedside

- Blood sugar — diabetic emergency with derangement in the septic toxic patient.
- Urine dipstick and analysis — myoglobinuria.

Laboratory-based investigations

- Blood cultures.
- Full blood count — a deranged white cell count with leucocytosis or leukopaenia.
- Raised C-reactive protein (CRP).
- Renal biochemistry — evidencing acute kidney injury.
- Elevated creatine kinase (CK) — evidence of associated muscle and tissue breakdown, rhabdomyolysis.
- Coagulation profile — evidence of disseminated intravascular coagulopathy (DIC).

Radiological investigations

- X-ray — gas in subcutaneous tissues.
- CT — subcutaneous air.
- MRI — extent of fascial necrosis seen which can guide the limits of debridement.

Other

- Biopsy — will aid in differentiating the affected tissue plane crucially, for example, fasciitis and cellulitis. A formal biopsy for histopathology and microbiology may be helpful to differentiate. A bed-side 'finger' test where a 2cm incision is made under local anaesthetic to deep fascial planes, and an assessment via finger palpation is made to see if it feels like the classical wet pus-filled cavity. This also provides a sample for frozen section, culture and Gram stain.
- Surgical exploration provides direct assessment of the tissues which will diagnose, but also delineate, the normal fascial plane from the diseased foul-smelling necrotising tissue.

5) What are the management priorities?

General measures

- Acute resuscitation to follow an 'airway, breathing, circulation, disability and exposure' approach, likely to include aggressive management of septic shock.
- Manage other comorbidities, in particular, diabetes.
- Nutritional support.

Pharmacological

- Specific antimicrobial therapy:
  - clindamycin is used to help suppress toxin production by *Streptococci*;
  - metronidazole is used for anaerobic organisms;
  - vancomycin may be required to cover methicillin-resistant *Staphylococcus aureus* (MRSA);
- Empiric antimicrobial therapy:
  - an example regime can be a carbapenem and clindamycin. For example, meropenem 1g or 25mg/kg Q8 hourly + clindamycin 600mg or 15mg/kg Q8 hourly;
  - depending on the suspected organisms or proven microbiological findings, the regime should be tailored, for example, to cover *Candida*, clostridial or *Vibrio* infection.

Surgical

- Early extensive surgical debridement.
- This may require repeated surgical visits for both surveillance and further debridement.
- The use of a vacuum-assisted wound closing device (VAC) can help support healing and recovery.

Special other

- Hyperbaric oxygen — used in anaerobic Gram-negative necrotising fasciitis.
- Intravenous immunoglobulin (IVIg). This may be of particular use for Group A *Streptococcus* necrotising fasciitis based on expert advice.
- Specialty teams likely to need alerting include:
  - microbiology and infectious diseases;
  - general surgery;
  - plastic surgery;
  - hyperbaric chamber.

Summary of Key Points

- Necrotising fasciitis is a life-threatening, rapidly progressive soft-tissue infection primarily involving the hypodermis and superficial fascia, with a high mortality rate of approximately 30%.
- It is associated with recent trauma and immunosuppressive states, for example, diabetes and chronic renal or liver disease.
- Clinical suspicion with early expedited surgery will allow for both prompt diagnosis and crucial management.
- The most common type accounting for 70% of cases is a polymicrobial Type I infection with anaerobic organisms.
- Prompt surgery with early antimicrobial therapy, including clindamycin to counter the toxin-producing *Streptococci* and anaerobic cover with carbapenems and metronidazole, provide a firm broad, initial foundation.

References

1. Young MH, Aronoff DM, Engleberg NC. Necrotizing fasciitis: pathogenesis and treatment. *Expert Rev Anti-infect Ther* 2005; 3(2): 279-94.
2. Misiakos EP, Bagias G, Patapis P, *et al.* Current concepts in the management of necrotizing fasciitis. *Front Surg* 2014; 1: 36.

SET 2

1) What are the pathological organisms involved in botulism and tetanus and how do they cause infection?

Botulism and tetanus are both toxin-mediated bacterial infections which affect the central nervous system.

Tetanus

- Infection by *Clostridium tetani*, an anaerobic Gram-positive toxin-producing bacterium. The toxin itself prevents pre-synaptic GABA inhibitory neurones from regulating motor neurone activity, causing the characteristic muscular spasms.
- Infection is from wound contamination with bacterial spores which are prevalent throughout nature, especially in soil.
- Vaccination programs have all but eradicated tetanus from the developed world, but the disease is still prevalent in countries without a vaccination program and in the immigrant population.

Botulism

- Infection by *Clostridium botulinum*, which is not a single uniform organism but a group of similar rod-shaped, Gram-positive, anaerobic and spore-forming organisms. They are distinguishable from each other only by the distinct (but similar) toxin that each species produces.

- Infection is possible via a number of routes:
    - enteral — ingestion of food containing the pre-formed toxin;
    - enteric — ingestion of the bacterial spores, then toxin production from within the gastrointestinal tract;
    - iatrogenic — a rare complication of the use of botulinum toxin for cosmetic reasons;
    - wound — infection with the bacteria or bacterial spore followed by *in vivo* toxin formation. It is most commonly associated with illicit drug use;
    - inhalational — aerosolisation of the toxin in a potentially weaponised form which could be used by terrorist organisations.

2) How might a patient with tetanus present?

C. tetani will not grow within healthy tissue so there needs to be a predisposing factor which usually includes a penetrating injury with or without a retained foreign body, localised ischaemia and coinfection with other bacteria. It is also important to note that the incubation period following spore inoculation is between 2 and 38 days (most commonly 7-10 days), so the initial injury may have healed or be unidentifiable. Generally, the shorter the incubation period, the more severe the infection and therefore the symptoms.

Generalised tetanus presents with the following symptoms and signs:

- Painful muscle spasms which occur periodically and may be triggered by sensory stimulation such as touch or loud noises.
- Trismus — the most common sign.
- Autonomic over-activity:
    - sweating;
    - irritability;
    - restlessness;
    - tachycardia and arrhythmias;

- cardiovascular instability;
- pyrexia.
- Dysphagia.
- Rigid abdominal musculature — mimicking a surgical abdomen.
- Periodic contraction of the thoracic or laryngeal musculature causing apnoea or upper airway obstruction/stridor.

It is important to note that there is no impairment in conscious level so patients are aware of the painful spasms which will contribute to the sympathetic response.

3) Outline the management of a patient with tetanus.

The management of acute tetanus is complex and should be undertaken by senior intensive care clinicians. The toxin binds irreversibly to the nervous system so the mainstay of treatment is supportive if this has already occurred, as well as to prevent further binding of any remaining free toxin. The goals of treatment are:

- Sedation and airway management — classically, sedation has been with high doses of benzodiazepine to control muscle spasms. Typically, patients may require hundreds of milligrams per day for a period of several weeks. Propofol may also be used either in isolation or in conjunction with benzodiazepines to reduce the dose and duration of their use. The quantity of sedative required contributes to the need for airway protection and mechanical ventilation. The period of ventilation is usually prolonged, so these patients almost universally require a tracheostomy to facilitate weaning.
- Control of muscle spasms — primarily with benzodiazepines but if this is insufficient, then the addition of neuromuscular blocking agents is indicated. There is some evidence for the use of baclofen via the intrathecal route but the required duration (average of 3 weeks in some studies) makes prolonged intrathecal access potentially problematic.

- Control of autonomic over-activity — this is best achieved with magnesium sulphate in doses equivalent to its use in pre-eclampsia. Trials have shown that it reduces the need for other cardiovascular stabilising drugs (calcium channel blockers) and reduces the dose of sedatives required to control spasm and pain but that it does not reduce the duration of mechanical ventilation.
- Control of toxin production by:
    - debridement of suspect wounds;
    - antibiotics, usually metronidazole.
- Control of unbound toxin — human tetanus immunoglobulin should be given to confer passive immunity and 'mop up' any unbound tetanus toxin before it can attach to the nervous system.
- Active immunisation — tetanus is one of only a few infections where immunity is not conferred following an acute infection; therefore, all patients with tetanus should be vaccinated with tetanus toxoid to a total of three doses 2 weeks apart starting as soon as the diagnosis is made.
- Supportive measures include:
    - early nutritional support as ongoing muscle spasms lead to a high energy requirement;
    - ventilator, pressure area and venous thromboembolism prophylaxis care bundles, due to the predicted long duration of intensive care unit admission;
    - physiotherapy as soon as the spasms cease, to reduce post-infection muscle loss and contractures.

4) What is the differential diagnosis of a patient presenting with botulism?

There are several neurological conditions which can present in a similar way to botulism, so these should be considered along with botulism if patients present with cranial nerve dysfunction (diplopia, dysphonia, dysarthria and dysphagia) followed by a descending motor weakness.

Such conditions include:

- The Miller-Fisher variant of Guillain-Barré syndrome — although this may present with ataxia as a predominant feature which botulism does not.
- A brainstem stroke — which may present with bulbar features.
- Other poisons/toxins — including neurotoxic snake envenomation, organophosphate poisoning, atropine overdose and heavy metal poisoning.
- Tick paralysis — rare outside of North America.
- Myasthenia gravis — usually presents with a longer prodrome involving weakness on repetitive movement and does not exhibit the autonomic features.

5) Outline the management of botulism.

General and medical management strategies are outlined below.

General

- Monitoring of respiratory function — patients should have serial forced vital capacity measurements plotted, with vigilance for a downwards trend. If the absolute level is below 10-15ml/kg, then the patient will usually require intubation and mechanical ventilation.
- Other indications for intubation may be impairment or loss of bulbar function and an inability to cough and clear saliva or respiratory tract secretions.
- Enteral nutrition via a nasogastric tube for patients unable to swallow.

Medical

- Antitoxin administration — the trivalent (against toxins A, B and E) equine antitoxin should be administered as soon as possible to bind free circulating toxin and prevent this from affecting the central nervous system. There is a high risk of anaphylaxis with this treatment and pre-treatment with steroids and antihistamines should be considered.

- Antibiotics — there is no evidence that antibiotics are beneficial in botulism, but they are usually administered especially in wound botulism where coinfection is likely. A common regime would be benzylpenicillin or metronidazole. It is important to note that aminoglycoside antibiotics should NOT be administered as they may potentiate the action of the toxin.

Summary of Key Points

- Both botulism and tetanus are bacterial illnesses which affect the central nervous system via toxin production.
- Tetanus infection can lead to prolonged intensive care unit admission, with all the associated complications.
- Tetanus infection does not confer immunity so all patients with tetanus should receive the standard vaccination course.
- Botulism is rare but may mimic other neurological conditions.
- Both conditions should have the appropriate antitoxin administered as soon as possible to bind free circulating toxin.

References

1.   Thwaites CL, Beeching NJ, Newton CR. Maternal and neonatal tetanus. *Lancet* 2015; 385: 362.

2.   Farrar JJ, Yen LM, Cook T, *et al*. Tetanus. *J Neurol Neurosurg Psychiatry* 2000; 69: 292.

3.   Engrand N, Guerot E, Rouamba A, Vilain G. The efficacy of intrathecal baclofen in severe tetanus. *Anesthesiology* 1999; 90: 1773.

4.   Thwaites CL, Yen LM, Loan HT, *et al*. Magnesium sulphate for treatment of severe tetanus: a randomised controlled trial. *Lancet* 2006; 368: 1436.

5.   Santos JI, Swensen P, Glasgow LA. Potentiation of *Clostridium botulinum* toxin aminoglycoside antibiotics: clinical and laboratory observations. *Pediatrics* 1981; 68: 50.

Eclampsia and HELLP syndrome

1) A) What is pre-eclampsia and can you classify the severity?

Pre-eclampsia

- Defined as hypertension (systolic of ≥140mmHg or diastolic of ≥90mmHg) after 20 weeks' gestation with significant proteinuria (urinary protein:creatinine ratio >30mg/mmol or 24-hour urine collection >300mg protein).

Severe pre-eclampsia

- Proteinuria plus severe hypertension (BP ≥160/110mmHg).
- OR moderate hypertension (140/90-159/109mmHg) plus any of the following:
  - severe headache;
  - visual disturbance such as flashing lights or blurring;
  - vomiting;
  - subcostal pain;
  - papilloedema;
  - clonus (≥3 beats);
  - liver tenderness;
  - thrombocytopenia (<100 × 10^9/L);
  - abnormal liver enzymes (ALT or AST >70 IU/L);
  - HELLP syndrome (haemolysis, elevated liver enzymes and low platelets).

Eclampsia

- Eclampsia is the occurrence of a seizure in association with pre-eclampsia.

B) What is HELLP syndrome and what are the complications?

- Haemolysis, elevated liver enzymes and low platelets:
  - evidence of haemolysis, falling haemoglobin (Hb) without overt bleeding, haemoglobinuria, elevated bilirubin (serum and urine), elevated LDH (>600 IU/L), blood film showing red cell fragments;
  - ALT/AST >70 IU/L;
  - thrombocytopenia, platelet count <100 x 10^9/L.
- Associated with pre-eclampsia and eclampsia (80% also have hypertension and proteinuria); the only definitive treatment is delivery of the placenta.
- Steroids do not alter progression but may be given to aid foetal lung maturity if the maternal condition is stable.
- Complications — the patient is at risk of renal failure, disseminated intravascular coagulation (DIC) and acute respiratory distress syndrome (ARDS); close monitoring and supportive management are required in a critical care environment.

2)   What are the associated risk factors?

Pregnancy-associated factors

classification

- Nulliparity.
- Multiple pregnancy.
- Donor insemination.
- Molar pregnancy.
- Chromosomal abnormalities.

Maternal factors

- >40 years.
- BMI ≥35kg/m² before pregnancy.
- Previous pre-eclampsia.

45

- Family history of pre-eclampsia.
- Booking diastolic blood pressure of 80mmHg or more.
- Associated diabetes, obesity, chronic hypertension and renal disease.
- Antiphospholipid antibodies and factor V Leiden.
- Pre-existing diabetes, hypertension, renal disease.
- A genetic contribution has been hypothesised but there is, as yet, no evidence to support the role of any particular gene.

Paternal factors

- First-time father.
- Family history of pre-eclampsia.

3) Describe the pathophysiology of pre-eclampsia.

Pre-eclampsia

- Several mechanisms have been proposed; however, it is generally accepted that poor invasion of the placental trophoblast cells results in failure of spiral artery dilatation, i.e. small high resistance vessels, instead of the normal large low resistance vessels which evolve as part of normal gestational physiology.
- The rigid vasoconstricted blood flow to the placenta causes hypoperfusion and hypoxia.
- In response, cytokines and inflammatory mediators are released into the maternal circulation.
- This triggers endothelial dysfunction causing increased vascular reactivity and permeability, and coagulation cascade activation resulting in oedema and microthrombi formation.

Eclampsia

- The mechanism of eclamptic seizures is not fully understood.

- Studies have shown that cerebral blood flow increases in both pre-eclampsia and eclampsia; however, in pre-eclampsia it is balanced by increased cerebrovascular resistance maintaining cerebral blood flow.
- Cerebral angiographic studies have demonstrated cerebral oedema and vasospasm. It is unclear whether the vasospasm is protective from the high arterial pressures or a pathological process.
- Cerebral oedema may be demonstrated on CT and MRI.

4) What investigations would you request and what would you expect to find?

Bedside

- Reagent strip urine testing — 1+ protein requires investigation.
- A urinary:protein creatinine ratio <30mg/mmol excludes significant proteinuria.
- 24-hour urine collection of ≥300mg which confirms and quantifies proteinuria.
- Non-invasive BP.

Laboratory — 6-hourly

- FBC for Hb and platelets.
- Liver biochemistry — elevated ALT/AST.
- Urea and electrolytes — transient renal impairment is common including hyperkalaemia.
- Coagulation screen — can be deranged, with disseminated intravascular coagulation (DIC) in extreme cases.
- Arterial blood gases — if indicated by clinical examination.

Radiological

- Chest X-ray if there is suspected pulmonary oedema.

- Transthoracic echocardiogram to check ventricular function in heart failure.

5) Outline the management of eclampsia

This is a critical obstetric emergency. Concurrent assessment, resuscitation and management should be carried out in an 'airway, breathing, circulation, disability, exposure' structure, with due diligence to the pregnancy including a left-lateral tilt or manual displacement of the uterus.

General

- Delivery of safe care with integrated close collaboration between midwifery, obstetric, anaesthetic, critical care and neonatology specialists is paramount.

Medical

- Treatment and prevention of further seizures using magnesium sulphate (the Collaborative Eclampsia Trial demonstrated greater effectiveness than phenytoin and diazepam), with a loading dose of 4g over 5 minutes followed by an infusion of 1g/hr for 24 hours. Recurrent seizures are treated with further boluses of 2g magnesium sulphate.
- Monitor for magnesium toxicity — diminished reflexes, low respiratory rate, low oxygen saturation and paralysis.
- Blood pressure control — aim for a controlled reduction to systolic <150mmHg and diastolic 80-100mmHg to prevent intracerebral haemorrhage.
- Moderate hypertension — oral labetalol is often the first choice; alternatives include nifedipine (caution with magnesium as there is a risk of toxicity) and methyldopa.

- Severe hypertension may require an IV infusion of labetalol or hydralazine (beware of hypotension with hydralazine) and institute invasive blood pressure monitoring.
- Hourly urine output and careful fluid balance.

Surgical

- Delivery of the foetus and placenta by caesarean section. General anaesthesia may be more difficult due to airway oedema but may be preferred to regional anaesthesia in view of reduced consciousness and coagulopathy.
- Attenuate the hypertensive response to laryngoscopy and extubation to avoid blood pressure surges causing intracranial haemorrhage.

6) As per the National Institute for Health and Care Excellence (NICE) guidance, which patients require a critical care referral?

Level 3 care

- Severe pre-eclampsia and/or needing ventilatory support.

Level 2 care

Step-down from level 3 or severe pre-eclampsia with any of the following complications:

- Eclampsia.
- HELLP syndrome.
- Haemorrhage.
- Hyperkalaemia.
- Severe oliguria.
- Requiring coagulation support.

- Requiring intravenous antihypertensive treatment.
- Initial stabilisation of severe hypertension.
- Evidence of cardiac failure.
- Abnormal neurology.

Summary of Key Points

- Eclampsia is a rare but avoidable cause of maternal mortality.
- The exact mechanism of eclamptic seizures is unknown but magnesium sulphate has been proven to be both preventative and the treatment of choice.
- NICE specifies the involvement of critical care for those with severe disease.

References

1. The Eclampsia Trial Collaborative Group. Which anticonvulsant for women with eclampsia? Evidence from the Collaborative Eclampsia Trial. *Lancet* 1995; 345(8963): 1455-63.

2. Visintin C, Mugglestone M, Almerie M, *et al*. Management of hypertensive disorders during pregnancy: summary of NICE guidance. *BMJ* 2010; 341: c2207.

3. Alladin A, Harrison M. Preeclampsia: systemic endothelial damage leading to increased activation of the blood coagulation cascade. *J Biotech Res* 2012; 4: 26-43.

4. Leslie D, Collis R. Hypertension in pregnancy. *BJA Education* 2015; 16(1): 33-7.

5. Allman K, Wilson I. *Oxford Handbook of Anaesthesia*, 2nd ed. Oxford University Press, 2016.

6. Hart E, Coley S. The diagnosis and management of pre-eclampsia. *Contin Educ Anaesth Crit Care Pain* 2003; 3(2): 38-42.

Respiratory weaning

1) A) Define respiratory weaning.

- Respiratory weaning is a gradual progressive reduction of mechanical ventilatory support until a patient is able to successfully breathe spontaneously.
- It involves a stepwise process:
  - readiness testing by evaluation of objective criteria to determine whether a patient can be safely switched from current ventilatory support to breathing without assistance, whether rapidly or gradually;
  - liberation from mechanical ventilation (extubation).
- Prolonged ventilation is associated with increased mortality, ventilator-associated pneumonias, lung injury and other complications, hence optimal weaning is preferable.

B) Classify the various types of weaning according to the time required to achieve liberation from a ventilator.

- Simple weaning (60% patients):
  - patients who can be extubated after demonstrating their spontaneous breathing is adequate to meet ventilatory requirements.
- Difficult weaning (30% patients):
  - patients who require up to three spontaneous breathing trials (SBTs) or as long as 7 days before extubation.
- Prolonged weaning (10% patients):
  - patients who exceed the timescale of difficult weaning and may require an individualised approach, often with the use of a tracheostomy which facilitates reduced sedation, reduced dead space and work of breathing, and aids secretion clearance.

2) A) Outline various clinical criteria used in assessing readiness for weaning.

- Improvement or resolution of the underlying cause of respiratory failure.
- Spontaneous respiratory efforts.
- Patient cooperative, pain-controlled, able to cough with minimal secretions, haemodynamically and metabolically stable, with optimal fluid balance.
- Adequate oxygenation:
  - PaO_2 >9kPa with FiO_2 <0.5 and PEEP <8cmH$_2$O.

B) Outline various physiological tests used to predict readiness for weaning.

- Minute ventilation <10-15L/min.
- Respiratory rate <35 breaths/min.
- Tidal volume <5ml/kg.
- Vital capacity >10ml/kg.
- Maximum inspiratory pressure (MIP) against occluded airway or negative inspiratory force (NIF) <-20cmH$_2$O (the more negative the better).
- Negative pressure that occurs 0.1 seconds after a spontaneous inspiratory effort (P0.1) <5cmH$_2$O.
- Rapid Shallow Breathing Index (RSBI, respiratory rate/tidal volume) <105 breaths/min/L.

C) What is a spontaneous breathing trial (SBT)?

An SBT is a test to determine whether a patient is likely to maintain adequate unassisted ventilation or is capable of weaning. There are two main methods:

- T-piece SBT:
  - disconnect the patient from mechanical ventilation and allow a period of spontaneous breathing via a T-piece;
  - duration of 30 minutes to 2 hours;
  - terminate as soon as signs of failure occur.
- Minimal ventilator support SBT:
  - either continuous positive airway pressure (CPAP) with tube compensation (automatic tube compensation [ATC] — Dräger; tube resistance compensation [TRC] — Hamilton) or low-level pressure support <8cmH$_2$O without PEEP;
  - duration of 30 minutes to 2 hours;
  - terminate as soon as signs of failure occur.

Signs of failure

- Clinical: agitation, anxiety, depressed conscious level, sweating, cyanosis, increased respiratory effort.
- Heart rate >20% baseline or >140 beats/min.
- Systolic blood pressure >20% baseline or >180mmHg or <90mmHg.
- Cardiac arrhythmias.
- RSBI >105 breaths/min/L.
- Respiratory rate >50% baseline or >35 breaths/min.
- Arterial oxygen saturation <90% or PaO$_2$ <8kPa on FiO$_2$ >0.5.
- PaCO$_2$ >6.5kPa or increased by >1kPa.
- pH <7.3 or fall by >0.07 units.

D) Outline various strategies for weaning.

- T-piece weaning:
  - involves disconnecting the patient from mechanical ventilation and allowing periods of spontaneous breathing via a T-piece for increasing lengths of time.
- Pressure support weaning:
  - involves periods of progressive reduction in pressure support for increasing lengths of time.

- Nurse-led weaning protocols have been shown to reduce the duration of mechanical ventilation.
- Sychronised intermittent mandatory ventilation (SIMV) mode is unsuitable for weaning.
- Other interventions also have proven benefit:
  - lung-protective ventilation;
  - daily interruptions to sedative infusions (sedation holds) — if associated with an SBT;
  - early physiotherapy and mobilisation;
  - conservative fluid management;
  - strategies to reduce ventilator-associated pneumonia (VAP care bundles).

3) A) Which factors require assessment to determine readiness for extubation?

- Successful spontaneous breathing trial.
- Adequate airway protection.
- Adequate airway patency.
- Adequate clearance of respiratory secretions.

B) What risk factors are associated with a high risk of extubation failure?

- Underlying cardiorespiratory disease.
- Neuromuscular disorders.
- Obesity.
- Positive fluid balance.
- Prolonged ventilation (>6 days).

C) What is the role of non-invasive ventilation (NIV) in weaning?

- NIV has proven efficacy in weaning certain patient groups, e.g. chronic obstructive pulmonary disease (COPD), acute cardiogenic pulmonary oedema.
- There may also be a role for extubation to immediate NIV subsequent to the failure of a spontaneous breathing trial and continued for at least 24 hours, with gradual weaning of NIV by increasing NIV-free time.

Summary of Key Points

- Respiratory weaning involves readiness testing using objective criteria, a rapid or gradual reduction in support (periods of T-piece spontaneous ventilation or reductions in pressure support) and eventual liberation from mechanical ventilation.
- Readiness for liberation from mechanical ventilation (extubation) can be assessed by the use of spontaneous breathing trials (SBTs) and adequacy of airway protection, patency and clearance of respiratory secretions. Weaning and extubation may also be facilitated by the use of lung-protective ventilation, sedation holds, early mobilisation, conservative fluid management, VAP care bundles, and the use of tracheostomies and non-invasive ventilation.

References

1. Gomersall C, *et al*. Mechanical ventilation: beyond BASIC. Hong Kong: The Department of Anaesthesia & Intensive Care, The Chinese University of Hong Kong, 2014.

2. Camporota L. Weaning and liberation from mechanical ventilation: clinical guideline, Version 1.0. London: Guy's and St Thomas' NHS Foundation Trust, 2014.

Acute liver failure

1) What is acute liver failure?

Acute liver failure is defined as new (<26 weeks) severe liver injury, with impaired synthetic function (INR >1.5) and encephalopathy. Fulminant hepatic failure is said to have developed if hepatic encephalopathy appears within 8 weeks of the onset of jaundice. Mortality remains high at 40-60%.

2) What is the epidemiology and aetiology of acute liver failure?

The overall incidence of acute liver failure is around 5.5 per million. Around 70% of those presenting with acute liver failure are female, with a median age at presentation of 38 years. In the developing world, viral disease is the most common cause, and in the developed world, drug-induced acute liver failure is more common. Paracetamol is the most common drug responsible for acute liver failure, with about half of all paracetamol overdose being unintentional.

The mnemonic VITAMIN can be used to further classify the aetiology (● Table 2.1).

Other causes include acute fatty liver of pregnancy, and HELLP syndrome/pre-eclampsia.

Table 2.1. The mnemonic VITAMIN to classify the aetiology of acute liver failure.

Vascular	Ischaemic hepatitis, Budd-Chiari syndrome
Infective	Hepatitis A, B, C, E viruses. Cytomegalovirus, *Herpes simplex*, parvovirus, Epstein-Barr
Trauma	Liver laceration
Autoimmune	Usually a cause of chronic liver failure, associated with other autoimmune conditions
Metabolic	Wilson's disease
Iatrogenic/idiopathic	Drug-induced including paracetamol, isoniazid, sulfa-containing drugs, antifungals
Neoplastic	Primary hepatic or metastatic lesions

3) Describe the clinical features of acute liver failure.

The clinical features of acute liver failure can be described using a systems-based approach.

Cardiovascular

Hypotension and hypovolaemia are common. Ascites occurs in up to 30% of patients, and bacterial peritonitis may present with shock refractory to fluid resuscitation.

Respiratory

Respiratory failure may develop and progress to ARDS.

Renal

Acute kidney injury is common, with a multifactorial aetiology including hypoperfusion, drug toxicity and acute tubular necrosis.

Neurological

Features of hepatic encephalopathy include confusion, depressed consciousness and seizures. Cerebral oedema may be seen.

Haematological

Impaired synthesis of coagulation factors may be accompanied by thrombocytopenia and haemolytic anaemia.

Metabolic

Hyperammonaemia and hypoglycaemia are common. Adrenal insufficiency can occur.

Immunological

Systemic inflammatory response syndrome (SIRS) is seen in up to 50% of cases. Nosocomial infection complicates the clinical course, with the respiratory and urinary tract being common sites of infection. Fungal infection is seen in up to 30% of patients.

4) How would you treat a patient with acute liver failure requiring intensive care unit admission?

The mainstay of treatment is the initiation of supportive measures.

Severe encephalopathy is managed by sedation, intubation and ventilation, with head-up positioning and control of $PaCO_2$ and volume status in order to minimise raised intracranial pressure and maintain cardiac output.

Noradrenaline is the preferred first-line vasopressor to maintain blood pressure. For those patients who fail to respond to a volume expansion and noradrenaline, vasopressin or terlipressin may potentiate the effects of noradrenaline.

If renal replacement therapy is required, continuous methods are preferred as they result in less haemodynamic instability.

N-acetylcysteine should be commenced for acute liver failure secondary to paracetamol overdose. It acts to replenish glutathione reserves, preventing accumulation of the toxic metabolite, N-acetyl-p-benzoquinone (NAPQI).

Viral-induced acute liver failure may be improved by the use of antiviral agents. Aciclovir has been successfully used to treat *Herpes simplex* virus hepatitis.

Pregnancy-induced acute liver failure is best treated by delivery of the foetus.

Liver transplantation is used for severe paracetamol-induced acute liver failure, as well as acute liver failure secondary to Wilson's disease. The modified King's College Criteria is most frequently used to predict those who would benefit from an emergency liver transplant.

Modified King's College Criteria

- pH <7.3; OR
- All three of:
  - INR >6.5;
  - creatinine >300μmol/L;
  - Grade III or IV encephalopathy.

Summary of Key Points

- Drug-induced liver failure is the most common aetiology in the developed world, with paracetamol being responsible for the majority of cases.
- Clinical features are wide-ranging and frequently necessitate organ support in a critical care environment.
- Treatment is supportive, with specific therapy depending on the cause.
- Liver transplantation should be considered in those with severe disease.

References

1. Punzalan C, Barry C. Acute liver failure: diagnosis and management. *J Intensive Care Med* 2016; 31(10): 642-53.

2. Blackmore L, Bernal W. Acute liver failure. *Clin Med* 2015; 15(5): 468-72.

Intensive care unit design and staffing

1) Are you aware of any guidelines pertaining to the building standards of an intensive care unit?

The Department of Health publishes "Health Care Building Notes" for all areas of primary and secondary care. There is a publication pertaining to the provision of intensive care unit services, which describes the services that should be adjacent to any intensive care unit as well as a prescriptive description of the make-up of the intensive care unit itself. The latter covers the overall layout of the unit — both the clinical and non-clinical spaces as well as minimum standards of provision of electrical sockets and square footage of bed spaces.

2) What do you understand by the term 'levels of critical care'? Can you define each level?

Levels of care pertain to the assistance a patient requires and where their care should be delivered. It also describes the number of organs which need to be supported to attain a level of care as well as the minimum ratio of nursing staff to provide this care.

The levels are defined by the Faculty of Intensive Care Medicine and the Intensive Care Society guidelines (● Table 2.2).

There is an unofficial 'Level 4', which is not described in the guidelines, but pertains to extraordinary levels of care in specialist units — for example, patients requiring extracorporeal membrane oxygenation (ECMO) necessitating additional staff to look after them.

Table 2.2. Levels of critical care defined by the Faculty of Intensive Care Medicine and the Intensive Care Society guidelines.

Level 0	Care which can be met with normal staffing of a ward in an acute hospital
Level 1	Patients with the potential to deteriorate or those who have stepped down from the critical care environment. Managed on an acute ward with input from the critical care team
Level 2	Patients requiring higher levels of care including single-organ system failure. Includes those stepping down from higher levels of care
Level 3	Patients requiring advanced respiratory support alone or basic respiratory support along with support of another organ system

3) What are the staffing ratios for medical and nursing staff on intensive care units?

Nursing staff ratios are based upon the levels of care as described above (● Table 2.3).

Additionally, there should be a supernumerary nursing coordinator and on larger intensive care units, supernumerary 'floating' nurses to assist with care and interventions.

Medical staff ratios are equally prescribed and there should be an intensive care resident junior doctor or advanced critical care practitioner for every 8 patients with an appropriate skill mix on any given shift. Similarly, it is recommended that each intensive care consultant supervises the care of between 8 and 15 patients.

Table 2.3. Nursing staff ratios for critical care.

Level 0	Care can be met by ward-based nursing staff
Level 1	Care is delivered by ward staff supported by critical care staff — outreach nursing and medical
Level 2	Care dictates a ratio of 1 nurse to 2 patients
Level 3	Care dictates a ratio of 1 nurse to 1 patient
Level 4	Care suggests a ratio of 2 nurses to 1 patient (one to look after the patient and one to look after the ECMO equipment)

4) If you were designing a hospital, where would you ideally site an intensive care unit?

Ideally, the intensive care unit would be located in the centre of the hospital. It requires easy access to a variety of other departments including but not limited to:

- The emergency department, acute medical unit and main theatres (elective and emergency).
- Radiology, including CT and MRI scanners.
- Haematology, biochemistry and microbiology laboratories including a blood bank.
- Pharmacy, for the provision of medicines and sterile services such as total parenteral nutrition.

Ideally, these would be all on the same floor with easy entrance and exits to the outside to facilitate admissions/transfers.

5) What additional staff are needed to support an intensive care unit?

A great number of professions support the intensive care unit:

- Pharmacists — review and reconcile the patient's own medication as well as advising on the addition of new medication. They are a vital link between pharmacy services for stock and the intensive care unit.
- Occupational therapists — support patients during rehabilitation and assess their need for ongoing specialist support, aids and services.
- Speech and language therapists — assist in patient communication for those patients who have ongoing ventilatory support needs and tracheostomies. They also assess the patient's ability to swallow safely as part of their weaning.
- Physiotherapists — from a musculoskeletal point of view, facilitate rehabilitation and the prevention of intensive care unit-acquired neuromyopathies. Also, they are key staff for respiratory assessment, therapy and weaning plans.
- Dietitians — assess and plan the patient's nutritional needs, either enteral or parenteral, and the provision of micronutrients for long-term patients.
- Chaplaincy, psychology and bereavement services — to support patients, their families and staff through critical illness and bereavement.
- Cleaners — to keep the intensive care unit free from pathogens. This includes specialist services for extraordinary cleaning after an infected patient has inhabited a cubical bed space.
- Secretarial/clerical staff — to organise the logistics and administration of intensive care unit patient movement, registration and discharge within a hospital's electronic database. They are integral to the provision and organisation of health care records and ICNARC data recording.

Summary of Key Points

- The Department of Health prescribes specific regulations for the provision of intensive care unit physical structures in its "Health Care Building Notes".
- Levels of care are linked to the requirement for organ support and staffing ratios.
- The intensive care unit is supported by a great many allied services and professionals.

References

1. Department of Health. Health Building Note 04-02 - Critical care units. Available from: https://www.gov.uk/government/publications/guidance-for-the-planning-and-design-of-critical-care-units.

2. Guidelines for the provision of intensive care services. The Faculty of Intensive Care Medicine and the Intensive Care Society, 2015. Available from: https://www.ficm.ac.uk/sites/default/files/gpics_-_ed.1_2015_v2.pdf.

Treatment withdrawal in the ICU

1) What categories of patients might be considered for treatment withdrawal?

- Imminent death — patients who deteriorate despite optimal therapy and are likely to die in the near future.
- Qualitative reasons — patients judged to have a poor neurological or functional outcome.
- Lethal conditions — patients with severe end-stage disease.

2) According to the GMC, which principles should guide end-of-life decision-making?

- Equalities and human rights — patients approaching the end of their life must be treated with the same dignity, respect, compassion and confidentiality as any other patient.
- Presumption in favour of prolonging life — not hastening death, although there is no absolute obligation to prolong life irrespective of the consequences for the patient and irrespective of the patient's views, if they are known or can be found out.
- Presumption of capacity — patients are presumed to have capacity until proven otherwise.
- Maximising capacity to make decisions — it is our duty to maximise our patient's ability to understand, retain and weigh the information we provide in order for them to reach a decision; if they are unable, which is common in the ICU, then the clinician must first consult any legal proxy such as a health and welfare lasting power of attorney who can make decisions on behalf of the patient; otherwise the clinician must decide, with help in ascertaining the patient's wishes provided by those close to the patient or an independent mental capacity advocate (IMCA).

- Overall benefit — the clinician must weigh any proposed benefits, burdens and risks associated with treatment options, incorporating both clinical and personal factors, in order to reach a conclusion regarding overall benefit to the patient.

3) What approach would you take in the process of treatment withdrawal on the ICU?

- Preparation — communication with the patient (if possible) and family, communication with and preparation of the multi-disciplinary team (including spiritual care if appropriate), an explanation on what to expect, and ideally moving the patient to a side room.
- Assessment of patient distress.
- Management of patient distress.
- Discontinuation of treatment and monitoring — rationalise non-comfort medications, stop vasopressors and inotropes, stepwise reduction in respiratory and other organ support.
- Bereavement support for families and potentially a debrief for staff.

4) List the common distressing symptoms patients may potentially encounter during the dying process, how they may be assessed or quantified and examples of management.

- Pain — assessment: Behavioural Pain Scale (BPS) or Critical Care Pain Observation Tool (CCPOT), clinical observation using objective signs; treatment: morphine and other opiates titrated to symptoms.
- Dyspnoea — assessment: Respiratory Distress Observation Scale (RDOS), clinical observation using objective signs; treatment: morphine and other opiates titrated to symptoms, anticholinergics for respiratory tract secretions.

- Agitation — assessment: Sedation-Agitation Score (SAS) or the Richmond Agitation Sedation Scale (RASS); treatment: benzodiazepines and other sedatives such as propofol titrated to symptoms.
- Delirium — assessment: Confusion Assessment Method for the Intensive Care Unit (CAM-ICU); treatment: haloperidol and non-pharmacological measures.
- Nausea and vomiting — clinical observation; treatment: antiemetics.

5) What particular areas of expertise may specialist palliative care teams provide to critical care?

- Assistance with treatment withdrawal decisions.
- Assessment and management of problematic symptoms.
- Facilitation of hospice or home care if appropriate.
- Continuity of care post-ICU discharge.

Summary of Key Points

- Treatment withdrawal is a valid consideration in patients facing imminent death, a poor outcome or with a lethal condition.
- End-of-life decision-making should incorporate equality, a presumption of prolonging life, maximising capacity and consideration of overall benefit.
- Withdrawal requires preparation, assessment and management of distressing symptomatology, discontinuation of treatment and monitoring and bereavement support.
- Symptoms requiring assessment and management include pain, dyspnoea, agitation, delirium, nausea and vomiting.
- Consider early referral to specialist palliative care teams.

References

1. Braganza MA, Glossop AJ, Vora VA. Treatment withdrawal and end-of-life care in the intensive care unit. *BJA Education* 2017; 17(12): 396-400.

2. Treatment and care towards the end of life: good practice in decision making. General Medical Council, 2010. Available from: http://www.gmc-uk.org/End_of_life.pdf _32486688.pdf.

3. Downar J, Delaney JW, Hawryluck L, Kenny L. Guidelines for the withdrawal of life-sustaining measures. *Intensive Care Med* 2016; 42(6): 1003-17.

SET 3

Management of life-threatening asthma

1) What is asthma?

Asthma is a chronic inflammatory disease of the airways which manifests itself as reversible airway obstruction in susceptible people who develop wheeze, cough, dyspnoea and chest tightness when provoked by a stimulus which may include cold weather, exertion, inter-current illness or airway manipulation. The inflammatory process is mediated by mast cells, eosinophils and T-lymphocytes.

2) How can asthma exacerbations be classified?

The British Thoracic Society (BTS) subclassifies acute exacerbations of asthma as follows:

- Moderate acute asthma — increased symptoms, peak expiratory flow rate (PEFR) >50-75% of best or predicted with no symptoms of acute severe asthma.
- Acute severe asthma — any one of:
    - PEFR 33-50% best or predicted;
    - respiratory rate ≥25/min;
    - heart rate ≥110/min;
    - inability to complete sentences in one breath.

- Life-threatening asthma — any one of the following in someone who satisfies the criteria for acute severe asthma:
  - altered conscious level;
  - exhaustion;
  - arrhythmia;
  - hypotension;
  - cyanosis;
  - silent chest; ✓
  - poor respiratory effort;
  - PEFR <33% best or predicted;
  - SpO_2 <92%;
  - PaO_2 <8kPa;
  - $PaCO_2$ 4.6-6kPa, i.e. 'normal'. ✗ not high
- Near fatal asthma — as for life-threatening asthma but with a rising $PaCO_2$ or requiring mechanical ventilation with high inflation pressures.

3)   What are the treatment priorities for acute life-threatening asthma?

The BTS has a guideline flow chart for the management of acute severe asthma. The intensive care doctor should be involved early in the management of these patients and it is important to ensure that simple measures have been instigated before more advanced management is considered. These include:

- Oxygen, aiming for oxygen saturations of 94-98%.
- A nebulised beta-2 agonist (driven by oxygen) — this is often enough to reverse the bronchospasm. Most commonly, salbutamol is used but there is no evidence that this is any better than terbutaline. Similarly, there is no apparent benefit from nebulised adrenaline instead of salbutamol.
- Steroids — either enteral prednisolone or intravenous hydrocortisone. Arguably this is the most important treatment and

although it will not have an immediate effect (it occurs at a cellular DNA level), there is good evidence to show that the anti-inflammatory effect reduces mortality, the duration of bronchospasm and the requirement for beta-2 agonists.

- Nebulised ipratropium bromide — synergistic with the beta-2 agonist, this acts to produce significantly greater bronchodilation leading to a faster recovery.
- An urgent chest X-ray to exclude pneumothorax — especially when using positive pressure ventilation.

More advanced measures should be delivered with the involvement of a senior intensive care medicine physician and may include:

- Intravenous magnesium sulphate — the evidence for this is somewhat contradictory with some studies showing that it provides no benefit. The consensus of the BTS is that a single dose of IV magnesium is safe, and MAY reduce intubation rates in patients with acute severe asthma. There is no role for nebulised magnesium sulphate in the management of acute severe or life-threatening asthma.
- Intravenous aminophylline — this may benefit a small proportion of patients with life-threatening exacerbations of asthma who have not responded to initial therapy. Unfortunately, the population who may benefit cannot be identified before the treatment, so an IV bolus (for those not already on oral theophylline) followed by an infusion should be considered.
- Intravenous salbutamol may be effective if the respiratory effort is so poor that the nebulised route is not delivering the drug to the bronchial levels where it is required to reverse bronchospasm.
- Ketamine, due to its known bronchodilatory properties, is the induction agent of choice should patients with life-threatening asthma need to be intubated. There are case reports of the use of low-dose boluses and infusions in unintubated patients, but the evidence is not yet strong enough for the BTS to recommend its routine use.

There are other potential therapies that are currently not recommended by the BTS for routine use in acute severe asthma based upon the evidence available. These include:

- Leukotriene receptor antagonists.
- Antibiotics empirically, unless there is good evidence for a bacterial infection (most infective exacerbations are likely to be viral in nature).
- Heliox, whilst useful in the management of acute upper airway obstruction, has no proven benefit in the smaller airways obstruction found in asthma.
- Nebulised DNase.
- Nebulised furosemide.

4) Who should you intubate for life-threatening asthma?

The decision to intubate patients with severe asthma can be a difficult one and senior clinicians should be involved if time allows. The indications for immediate intubation and mechanical ventilation include:

- Respiratory failure — characterised by a reducing respiratory rate, lowering of oxygen saturation or rising $PaCO_2$ in a patient who is clearly not responding to treatment.
- Reduced conscious level which may be as a result of exhaustion, hypoxaemia or hypercapnia.

The most experienced clinician present should intubate the patient with the widest possible internal diameter of endotracheal tube to maximise expiratory flow.

5) What would be your mechanical ventilatory strategy for patients with life-threatening asthma?

The strategy for ventilating asthmatics with severe bronchospasm involves:

- Efforts to prevent (or at least recognise) dynamic hyperinflation — so called 'gas trapping', where the patient is not permitted to fully exhale, leading to each breath adding a small volume of gas that remains inside the lungs. Over time, this causes distension and eventually leads to over-distended lungs which then cannot be ventilated. Any ventilated asthmatic who deteriorates in terms of hypoxaemia, hypotension or ventilator alarms pertaining to high pressures should be immediately disconnected from the ventilator and have their chest mechanically decompressed to rule out gas trapping as the cause. The strategy to prevent it occurring includes:
  - low respiratory rates — with long expiration times — to allow the lungs to fully empty;
  - low tidal volumes;
  - limiting plateau pressures to <30cmH$_2$O;
  - judicious use of PEEP — although controversial, PEEP may be detrimental and extrinsic PEEP should be below the level of intrinsic PEEP (although this may be a difficult measure with severe widespread bronchospasm). If in doubt, then extrinsic PEEP should be avoided in the first instance.

  These measures may lead to hypercapnia, but this should be permitted (as long as the pH is acceptable) in order to maintain oxygenation, full expiration and prevent hyperinflation.
- Close attention should be paid with regards to changes in compliance. If pressure-controlled ventilation is being utilised, then once the bronchospasm breaks the previously high pressures required to adequately ventilate patients, this may now lead to excessive tidal volumes and volutrauma.

Summary of Key Points

- Asthma kills people and should be respected.
- Every intensive care doctor should be familiar with the diagnosis and severity of acute asthma.
- The advanced management of acute severe and life-threatening asthma should be led by a senior intensive care physician and they should be clear on the evidence for each treatment.
- The decision to intubate patients can be a difficult one and careful judgement is required along with a recognition of the speed with which these patients can deteriorate.
- Patients who are intubated and become hypoxic, hypotensive or whose ventilator starts alarming for high pressure/low volume, should immediately be disconnected from the ventilator and their chest mechanically emptied to rule out gas trapping as the cause.

References

1. British Thoracic Society/SIGN guideline on the management of asthma, 2016. Available from: https://www.brit-thoracic.org.uk/document-library/clinical-information/asthma/btssign-asthma-guideline-2016/.

2. Rodrigo GJ, Nannini LJ. Comparison between nebulized adrenaline and beta2 agonists for the treatment of acute asthma. A meta-analysis of randomized trials. *Am J Emerg Med* 2006; 24(2): 217- 22.

3. Rowe BH, Spooner C, Ducharme F, *et al*. Corticosteroids for preventing relapse following acute exacerbations of asthma. *Cochrane Database Syst Rev* 2007; Issue 3.

4.   Stoodley RG, Aaron SD, Dales RE. The role of ipratropium bromide in the emergency management of acute asthma exacerbation: a metaanalysis of randomized clinical trials. *Ann Emerg Med* 1999; 34(1): 8-18.

5.   Kew KM, Kirtchuk L, Michell CI. Intravenous magnesium sulfate for treating adults with acute asthma in the emergency department. *Cochrane Database Syst Rev* 2014; Issue 5.

6.   Parameswaran K, Belda J, Rowe BH. Addition of intravenous aminophylline to beta2-agonists in adults with acute asthma. *Cochrane Database Syst Rev* 2000; Issue 4.

Myasthenia gravis and myasthenic crisis

1) What is myasthenia gravis?

Myasthenia gravis (MG)

- A chronic, autoimmune disorder of the postsynaptic membrane of the nicotinic neuromuscular junction (NMJ) in skeletal muscle.
- Neuromuscular transmission is impaired by circulating autoantibodies to nicotinic acetylcholine receptors (AChR) and associated proteins.
- Characterised by muscle weakness that increases with exercise (fatigue) and improves on rest.
- Most patients enjoy a normal quality of life but 15-20% will have a myasthenic crisis requiring ventilatory support.
- Severity ranges from mild ptosis to bulbar and respiratory weakness requiring ventilatory support.

2) Please describe the Myasthenia Gravis Foundation of America clinical classification (● Table 3.1), and state which patients require critical care intervention.

Table 3.1. Myasthenia Gravis Foundation of America clinical classification.
Class I   Any eye muscle weakness; possible ptosis; all other muscle strength is normal
Class II   Mild weakness of other muscles; may have eye muscle weakness of any severity
Class III   Moderate weakness of other muscles; may have eye muscle weakness of any severity
Class IV   Severe weakness of other muscles; may have eye muscle weakness of any severity
Class V   Intubation needed to maintain airway

- As per the classification, patients with Classes IV and V MG will require critical care input.

3) What patient groups and risk factors are associated with myasthenia gravis?

- This is an uncommon condition, with a worldwide prevalence of 100-200 per million.
- It is more common in women who tend to present during childbearing years; the median age in men is in the seventh decade.
- There is a genetic component, possibly major histocompatibility complex (MHC)-meditated.
- The presence of autoimmune disease in the patient or family members.

4) Briefly outline the pathophysiology of myasthenia gravis.

The pathophysiology is not fully understood and research is ongoing. Antibodies to the AChR are important but other antibody types have been discovered. AChR antibodies:

- Block the attachment of ACh decreasing the number of functional receptors.
- Increase the receptor degradation rate.
- Cause complement-induced damage to the NMJ.

Some patients lack AChR antibodies but may have antibodies for other targets, for example, muscle-specific tyrosine kinase, low-density lipoprotein receptor-related protein (LRP4), agrin, collagen Q and cortactin.

70% of patients with MG have thymic follicular hyperplasia and 10% have thymoma.

5) What are the clinical features of MG?

MG commonly presents with:

- Ptosis (drooping eyelids).
- Diplopia (double vision).
- Dysphagia (oropharyngeal weakness).
- Dysarthria.
- Proximal limb weakness.
- Shortness of breath.

6) What investigations would you order and what might you see for someone suspected of having MG?

Laboratory-based investigations

- 80-90% have detectable autoantibodies to the nicotinic AChR; another 3-7% have antibodies against muscle-specific tyrosine kinase (MuSK).

Radiological

- Consider imaging, specifically CT chest — to detect thymoma.

Other

- Serial pulmonary function tests.
- Electrophysiology — repetitive nerve stimulation shows a decremental response.

7) What are the management priorities in a myasthenic crisis?

This is a potential critical emergency. Concurrent assessment, resuscitation and management should be carried out in an 'airway, breathing, circulation, disability, exposure' structure, with due diligence to call up appropriate skilled personnel, equipment and drugs.

Specific management priorities are outlined below.

General measures

- Myasthenic crises are often precipitated by infections. Recognition can be delayed due to steroid treatment.

Medical pharmacological

- Anticholinesterase — regular oral pyridostigmine.

Surgical

- Consider a thymectomy once the patient is stabilized, as there is RCT evidence showing a benefit of thymectomy for MG patients with Class IV disease and AChR antibodies.

Special other

- Intravenous immunoglobulin.
- Plasma exchange.

Preparation for elective procedures

- Function should be assessed by a neurologist and optimised before any elective procedure; those with bulbar and respiratory symptoms may require postoperative ventilation.
- Continuation of oral anticholinesterase treatment is important. Consider nasogastric feeding if the oral route is compromised.
- If muscle relaxation is required to facilitate intubation, then depolarising neuromuscular blocking (NMB) drugs, e.g. suxamethonium, should be avoided as they can cause phase II block.
- Non-depolarising NMB drugs should be avoided but short/medium-acting agents, e.g. atracurium, rocuronium, can be used at 10-20% of normal dose.

Indications for mechanical ventilation

- Forced vital capacity (FVC) ≤15ml/kg.
- Negative inspiratory force (NIF) ≤20cmH$_2$O.

8) What key drugs are of interest in MG (● Table 3.2)?

Table 3.2. Drugs used in MG.

Drug	Interaction	Comment
Non-depolarising neuromuscular blocking agents	Increased sensitivity	Use 10-20% normal dose, short/medium-acting agents only and monitor effect
Depolarising NMB drugs (suxamethonim)	Delayed onset	Delayed recovery in patients with esterase deficiency (e.g. post-plasmapheresis). No reports of harm with 1.5mg/kg
Inhalational anaesthetics	Reduce neuromuscular transmission	Can therefore avoid NMB drugs
Propofol	No clinical effect on neuromuscular transmission	Can deliver total intravenous anaesthesia (TIVA) without affecting neuromuscular function
Drugs eliminated using esterases	Prolonged effect and risk of toxicity	Suxamethonium, remifentanil, mivacurium, ester local anaesthetics
Acetylcholinesterase inhibitors, e.g. neostigmine	Risk of cholinergic crisis if used to reverse NMB drugs	Use atracurium or rocuronium if an NMB drug is required
Antibiotics	Neuromuscular blocking effects may become important	Avoid aminoglycosides, e.g. gentamicin

Summary of Key Points

- Myasthenia gravis is a chronic, autoimmune, IgG-mediated disorder of the postsynaptic membrane of the neuromuscular junction (NMJ), specifically at nicotinic acetylcholine receptors (AChR) and associated proteins.
- Most patients have a good quality of life and normal life span due to prompt diagnosis and good management.
- Care must be taken to avoid precipitating myasthenic or cholinergic crises which will require critical care involvement.

References

1. Myasthenia gravis. Summary - Best Practice, 30 April 2017. Available from: http://bestpractice.bmj.com/best-practice/monograph/238/highlights/summary.html.
2. Allman K, Wilson I. *Oxford Handbook of Anaesthesia*, 2nd ed. Oxford University Press, 2016.
3. Phillips L. The epidemiology of myasthenia gravis. *Sem Neurol* 2004; 24(1): 17-20.
4. Thavasothy M, Hirsch N. Myasthenia gravis. *Contin Educ Anaesth Crit Care Pain* 2002; 2(3): 88-90.
5. Wolfe G, Kaminski H, Aban I, *et al*. Randomized trial of thymectomy in myasthenia gravis. *N Engl J Med* 2016; 375(6): 511-22.

Anticoagulation for renal replacement therapy and heparin-induced thrombocytopenia

1) What methods of anticoagulation can be utilised in renal replacement therapy?

- No anticoagulation if the patient is auto-anticoagulated (coagulopathy and/or low platelets).
- Systemic delivery:
  - unfractionated heparin;
  - low-molecular-weight heparin;
  - heparinoids, e.g. danaparoid;
  - direct thrombin inhibitors, e.g. argatroban;
  - prostacyclin, e.g. Flolan®.
- Regional delivery:
  - citrate — chelates calcium, thus inhibiting platelet aggregation and coagulation. A systemic calcium infusion is necessary in order to avoid hypocalcaemia;
  - heparin with protamine.

2) Briefly outline the pathophysiology of heparin-induced thrombocytopenia (HIT).

- HIT is a life- and limb-threatening pathological syndrome occurring when heparin-dependent IgG antibodies bind to heparin/platelet factor 4 complexes to activate platelets and produce a hypercoagulable state with venous and arterial thrombosis.
- The resulting thrombocytopenia and thrombosis with HIT typically develops 5-10 days after administration of unfractionated heparin (incidence 1-5%), low-molecular-weight heparin (incidence <1%), and, very rarely, fondaparinux.
- The highest incidence is in patients who receive heparin post-surgery or trauma.
- Women have a 1.5-2-fold increased risk of HIT compared with men.

3) Describe a commonly used clinical prediction tool for HIT.

- The Warkentin (4Ts) Probability Scale is the most evaluated HIT scoring tool to date.
- Points are given from 0-2 for four categories:
  - magnitude of thrombocytopenia;
  - timing of onset of decrease in platelet count (or other sequelae of HIT);
  - thrombosis or other sequelae;
  - other causes for the decrease in platelet count.
- A low score (0-3) indicates a <1% probability of HIT.
- An intermediate score (4-5) approximates a 10% probability of HIT.
- A high score (6-8) approximates a 50% probability of HIT.

4) How is HIT diagnosed?

Compatible clinical picture

- History of heparin use and timing, recent surgery or trauma, lack of other conditions or drugs causing thrombocytopenia.
- Symptoms and signs of recent venous or arterial thromboembolic events.
- Acute systemic reaction:
  - fever;
  - chills;
  - tachycardia;
  - hypertension;
  - dyspnoea;
  - cardiopulmonary arrest.

Laboratory tests

- Full blood count — reduced platelet count.
- Clotting — exclude coagulopathy; disseminated intravascular coagulation may be induced in 10-20% patients with HIT.

- Heparin-dependent platelet activating heparin-induced thrombocytopenia (HIT) antibodies — patients with an intermediate/high 4Ts score should undergo testing for HIT antibodies.

Imaging

- Doppler ultrasonography — for suspected arterial or deep venous thromboembolism.
- Computed tomography pulmonary angiography (CTPA) or ventilation-perfusion scanning (V/Q scan) — for suspected pulmonary embolism.
- Computed tomography or magnetic resonance imaging venography — for suspected cerebral venous thrombosis.

5) How is confirmed HIT managed?

- Stopping the heparin.
- If warfarin has been started, commence oral or intravenous vitamin K.
- Consider starting a non-heparin anticoagulant for treatment or prevention of thromboembolism, for example:
  - argatroban;
  - bivalirudin;
  - danaparoid;
  - fondaparinux may be used in patients who have never had fondaparinux-associated HIT.

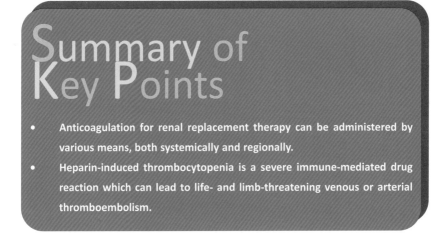

Summary of
Key Points

- Anticoagulation for renal replacement therapy can be administered by various means, both systemically and regionally.
- Heparin-induced thrombocytopenia is a severe immune-mediated drug reaction which can lead to life- and limb-threatening venous or arterial thromboembolism.

References

1. Linkins L-A. Heparin induced thrombocytopenia. *BMJ* 2015; 350: g7566.

Influenza

1) A) What kind of viruses cause seasonal influenza?

- Influenza viruses are part of the orthomyxoviridae family of RNA viruses.
- Of the three types of influenza virus, A, B, and C, seasonal influenza is most often caused by Type A or B.

B) What do we mean by influenza epidemics and pandemics, and what are they caused by?

- Influenza epidemics are seasonal (particularly during the winter months). Localized infection outbreaks caused by minor changes in the viral NA or HA glycoproteins, termed antigenic drift, cause less severe disease in individuals who have been exposed to the antecedent virus.
- Influenza pandemics occur when a Type A virus undergoes a major change, termed antigenic shift, due to the acquisition of new gene segments creating an influenza strain to which the majority of the population do not have immunity, causing rapid and worldwide spread.
- Seasonal influenza viruses may contribute to the emergence of a pandemic virus and once a pandemic virus has been established, it can become a seasonal virus.

2) A) What are the clinical manifestations of the influenza virus infection?

In most patients, influenza presents as a non-specific, self-limiting, uncomplicated, acute illness of short duration (typically less than a week):

- Fever.
- Cough — which can be severe and may last 2 or more weeks.

- Headache.
- Pharyngitis.
- Rhinorrhoea.
- Myalgia.
- Arthralgia.
- Fatigue.
- Vomiting and diarrhoea.

B) List a few differential diagnoses.

- Community-acquired pneumonia.
- Hospital-acquired pneumonia.
- Severe acute respiratory infection.
- Exacerbations of chronic lung disease, e.g. asthma, COPD.
- Generalised sepsis.
- Encephalopathy, encephalitis, transverse myelitis, aseptic meningitis, Guillain-Barré syndrome.
- Myocarditis.
- Rhabdomyolysis.

C) Outline the complications that can occur with influenza infection.

Complications include:

- Respiratory system, e.g. viral pneumonia, ARDS.
- Central nervous system, e.g. encephalitis.
- Cardiovascular system, e.g. myocarditis.
- Musculoskeletal system, e.g. myositis, rhabdomyolysis.
- Obstetric complications, e.g. premature labour, miscarriage, stillbirth.
- Sepsis and multi-organ failure.
- Secondary bacterial infections:
  - pneumonia, e.g. *Streptococcus pneumoniae, Staphylococcus aureus, Haemophilus influenzae.*

- septicaemia and other invasive bacterial infections, e.g. *Streptococcus, Neisseria meningitidis, Staphylococcus aureus.*
- Secondary fungal infections, e.g. *Aspergillus.*

D) Which groups of patients are at particularly high risk of severe illness and death?

High-risk groups include:

- Pregnant women, including up to 2 weeks post-partum.
- Children younger than 5 years.
- Elderly over 65 years.
- Those with chronic medical conditions such as:
    - HIV/AIDS and other conditions causing immunosuppression;
    - respiratory disease, e.g. asthma, COPD, cystic fibrosis;
    - neurological disease, e.g. neuromuscular, neurocognitive, seizure disorders;
    - renal disease, e.g. chronic kidney disease (CKD) requiring dialysis or transplantation;
    - liver disease, e.g. cirrhosis;
    - cardiovascular disease;
    - diabetes mellitus;
    - morbidly obese (BMI >40).
- Those at increased risk of exposure such as healthcare workers.

3) Which laboratory investigations aid in establishing a diagnosis of influenza infection?

- Appropriate diagnostic samples should be obtained as soon as influenza is suspected.
- The gold standard method for detecting influenza viruses is to send samples for detection of viral RNA by reverse transcription followed by PCR. Potential samples include:
    - nose and throat swabs;
    - nasopharyngeal and tracheal aspirates;

- bronchial washings (endotracheal tube aspirate; non-directed bronchial lavage; bronchoalveolar lavage), if there is clinical suspicion of viral lower respiratory infection, as upper respiratory tract samples may be negative;
- lumbar puncture with CSF for detection of influenza in patients suspected of CNS complications;
- other samples for bacterial and fungal complications, e.g. respiratory tract secretions, blood cultures, urine for pneumococcal testing.
- Viral load estimation may help in determining antiviral effect.
- Laboratory testing for antiviral resistance may also be available.

4) A) How would you approach the treatment of patients with severe illness due to influenza?

- General supportive care with organ support.
- Antiviral therapy with neuraminidase inhibitors should be started empirically before a virological diagnosis has been obtained:
  - oseltamivir (Tamiflu®) usually for immunocompetent patients;
  - zanamivir (Relenza®) usually for immunocompromised patients;
  - local protocols will determine which agent is first-line depending on the dominant circulating influenza virus;
  - intravenous zanamivir is available on a named patient basis for the critically ill and those unable to tolerate the enteral route;
  - treatment duration varies on a case-by-case basis, but may be extended beyond 10 days in the critically ill and severely immunocompromised.
- There is evidence for a reduction in symptoms and disease severity and mortality, particularly if antivirals are started within 48 hours of illness onset.
- Corticosteroids are not recommended for treating complicated influenza, but should not be withheld if required for another indication.

B) Which groups of patients are at risk of antiviral resistance?

- Severely immunocompromised.
- Patients who develop influenza whilst, or shortly after, receiving antiviral prophylaxis.
- Contacts of known resistance cases.
- Patients who have changed antiviral therapy.
- Patients who clinically deteriorate during antiviral therapy.

5) A) How does human-to-human transmission of the influenza virus occur?

- The influenza virus is present in the respiratory secretions of infected persons.
- Transmission occurs primarily by direct and indirect contact with large-particle respiratory droplets, following coughing and sneezing.
- It is possible that transmission may also occur through short-range aerosolisation of small-particle droplets.

B) Outline the general principles of influenza virus infection prevention and control.

- Follow local infection prevention and control policies.
- Staff vaccination program.
- Infected patients should be placed in single rooms for respiratory isolation, or else cohorted, if possible.
- Use droplet and contact precautions:
  - good hand hygiene;
  - daily room cleaning;
  - surfaces touched by patients cleaned thrice daily;
  - personal protective equipment (PPE) should be worn and removed appropriately by staff and visitors within 2m of a patient with suspected or confirmed influenza:
    - plastic apron;

- ■ disposable gloves;
- ■ surgical mask;
- ■ eye protection if there is a risk of eye exposure;
- - terminal cleaning following discharge.
- Aerosol-generating procedures should be avoided if possible, otherwise the following must be used:
  - - FFP3 face mask or respirator (fit tested and checked);
  - - disposable gloves;
  - - fluid-repellent gown;
  - - eye protection.
- Mitigate the risk of aerosol-generating devices such as ventilators and humidifiers according to manufacturers' instructions:
  - - bacterial/viral filters;
  - - closed tracheal suctioning.
- Continue precautions for 24 hours after resolution of fever and respiratory signs and symptoms, although longer may be required in the immunocompromised.

Summary of Key Points

- Seasonal influenza is most often caused by Type A or B influenza RNA viruses, with pandemics caused by Type A.
- Influenza usually presents with a non-specific acute respiratory illness, but may progress to multisystem complications and secondary bacterial and fungal infections in some patients, particularly those at high risk.
- The gold standard diagnosis is by PCR detection of influenza viral RNA from appropriate samples.

- Treatment includes general supportive care and early empirical antiviral therapy in suspected cases.
- Robust infection prevention and control measures are important to contain further infection spread.

References

1.   Public Health England. Seasonal influenza: guidance for adult critical care units. London: PHE Publications, 2017. Available from: https://www.gov.uk/government/uploads/system/uploads/attachment_data/file/635596/adult__seasonal_influenza_critical_care_guidance.pdf.

2.   Johnstone C, Hall A, Hart IJ. Common viral illnesses in intensive care: presentation, diagnosis, and management. *Contin Educ Anaesth Crit Care Pain* 2014; 14(5): 213-9.

Diabetic emergencies — diabetic ketoacidosis (DKA) and hyperosmolar hyperglycaemic state (HHS)

1) What are common precipitants for diabetic emergencies?

There is almost always an identifiable event that has led a patient with normally stable diabetes to have a hyperglycaemic diabetic emergency:

- The most common underlying cause is an infective process — typically within the respiratory or urinary tract.
- Failure to take their normal insulin or inadequate dosing of insulin is another common cause.
- Diabetic ketoacidosis (DKA) can be the first presentation of Type 1 diabetes in a patient who has therefore not yet been exposed to exogenous insulin.
- Drugs taken for other reasons — particularly steroids — can precipitate hyperglycaemia by increasing insulin resistance.
- Non-infective major illnesses with a stress response such as a myocardial infarction or stroke.

2) How do patients with DKA or HHS present?

Both DKA and HHS patients will present with a short history of general deterioration or symptoms of the underlying precipitating cause as well as specific hyperglycaemic/metabolic symptoms. The period of decline is often more rapid in DKA than in HHS:

- Polydipsia and polyuria — driven by the osmotic diuretic effect of elevated serum glucose level exceeding the ability of the nephron to reabsorb all of the glucose.
- Lethargy or altered conscious level ranging from acute confusion to coma — this is related to the plasma osmolality, >320mosmol/kg, causing obtundation; therefore, this is more common in HHS where osmolality levels are generally higher.

- Nausea and vomiting, which then contributes further to dehydration.
- Dehydration — evident by tachycardia, possible hypotension, dry mucous membranes, cool peripheries, delayed capillary refill, increased skin turgor and renal dysfunction.
- Patients with DKA may also show signs of metabolic acidosis by attempting to compensate with the respiratory system — Kussmaul respiration. The ketones may be detectable on their breath with the presence of a 'fruity odour'.
- Abdominal pain occurs more frequently in DKA than HHS and may be as a result of ileus secondary to metabolic acidosis. It is important to ensure that there is not an underlying intra-abdominal pathology which is the trigger for DKA in those patients who present with abdominal pain, e.g. acute appendicitis.
- Both groups will have an elevated serum glucose level, but this is generally at a higher level in HHS than in DKA.

3) What are the main management priorities for patients with DKA or HHS?

Management priorities in DKA and HHS include:

- Treat the precipitating cause.
- Dehydration is the most important factor to correct in both DKA and HHS, and correction of circulating volume takes precedence over correcting the serum glucose levels. Generally, HHS patients will be more dehydrated than DKA patients due to the higher glucose levels exacerbating osmotic diuresis, as well as the longer prodrome to presentation in this group. Typically, patients with DKA will be 3-6L negative and patients with HHS will be 8-10L negative:
  - if hypotensive, then fluid boluses should be given to restore perfusion;
  - resuscitate with a crystalloid such as 0.9% sodium chloride;

- the optimal rate of fluid replacement is 15-20ml/kg/hr for the first 2 hours followed by a rate reduction. The overall fluid amount should not exceed 50ml/kg in the first 4 hours;

- after this, the ongoing rate of fluid resuscitation should be guided by the volume status of the patient judged on clinical parameters and by any electrolyte abnormalities.

● The patient is likely to have significant potassium depletion due to renal and gastrointestinal losses. The initial serum potassium may be high due to the acidosis and dehydration but will quickly drop once fluid resuscitation and correction of the acidosis occurs. Potassium replacement should therefore start in combination with the insulin therapy, as this will further drop the serum potassium as insulin promotes the intracellular uptake of potassium. The potassium level should be measured frequently in the first 6-8 hours of treatment.

● Insulin therapy should be commenced after fluid resuscitation and with careful consideration of the serum potassium, with a fixed rate intravenous insulin infusion (FRIII) commenced at 0.1 units/kg/hr. The insulin primarily acts to prevent hepatic production of glucose rather than peripheral glucose utilisation. Hourly monitoring of ketones (e.g. bedside 3-beta-hydroxybutyrate) and serum glucose levels is essential (with the aim of reducing ketones by 0.5mmol/L/hr), with 2-hourly measurement of pH, potassium and bicarbonate over the first 6 hours of treatment. Intravenous dextrose must be added to the maintenance fluid once the glucose reaches <14mmol/L.

4) What complications may ensue as a result of mismanagement of the hyperglycaemic state?

Common complications

● Hypoglycaemia — as a result of overshooting on insulin therapy or failing to recognise the need to add IV glucose as an energy substrate once the serum glucose level is <14mmol/L.

● Hypokalaemia — failure to recognise that the body is in a state of overall potassium deficit despite the initial serum level being normal or high.

Rarer complications

- Pulmonary oedema — usually non-cardiogenic in nature due to the rapid decline in plasma oncotic pressure associated with the correction of hyperglycaemic states — this allows an increase in extracellular lung water which can manifest as hypoxaemia with decreased lung compliance.
- Cerebral oedema — more common in children and as a complication of HHS, where the initial serum osmolality is higher, and too rapid a correction can precipitate fluid shifts and cerebral oedema. The first symptom of this is usually headache and this should be taken seriously in the context of treating HHS, as unrecognised it has a high morbidity and mortality.

5) When should patients with DKA who require critical care admission be restarted on their normal subcutaneous insulin regime?

There are no hard and fast rules; however, the following points should be taken into consideration:

- Subcutaneous (SC) insulin should be started before intravenous (IV) insulin is discontinued.
- The patient should be able to eat and drink normally when restarting their normal SC insulin.
- In HHS, the serum glucose should be less than 13.9mmol/L.
- In DKA, the serum glucose should be less than 11mmol/L.
- Other considerations in DKA:
    -   pH >7.30;
    -   serum anion gap <12mmol/L;
    -   serum bicarbonate >15mmol/L.

Summary of Key Points

- There is almost always an underlying precipitant to DKA/HHS — look for it.
- DKA and HHS present in a similar manner with a higher glucose level in HHS.
- The main issues in treating DKA/HHS are treating the precipitating cause, correction of circulating volume and total body potassium depletion, and insulin therapy.
- Hypoglycaemia and hypokalaemia are common complications of poor treatment of DKA/HHS.
- SC insulin should be restarted in conjunction with tapering IV insulin once the patient has recovered from the metabolic derangement caused by the hyperglycaemic state.

References

1.   Wachtel TJ, Silliman RA, Lamberton P. Prognostic factors in the diabetic hyperosmolar state. *J Am Geriatr Soc* 1987; 35: 737.

2.   Daugirdas JT, Kronfol NO, Tzamaloukas AH, Ing TS. Hyperosmolar coma: cellular dehydration and the serum sodium concentration. *Ann Intern Med* 1989; 110: 855.

3.   Kitabchi AE, Umpierrez GE, Miles JM, Fisher JN. Hyperglycemic crises in adult patients with diabetes. *Diabetes Care* 2009; 32: 1335.

4.   Brun-Buisson CJ, Bonnet F, Bergeret S, *et al*. Recurrent high-permeability pulmonary edema associated with diabetic ketoacidosis. *Crit Care Med* 1985; 13: 55.

5.   Kerr DE, Wenham T, Munir A. Endocrine problems in the critically ill 1: diabetes and glycaemic control. *BJA Education* 2017; 17(11): 370.

Abdominal compartment syndrome

1) Can you define intra-abdominal hypertension (IAH) and abdominal compartment syndrome?

A normal intra-abdominal pressure is thought to be between 5-7mmHg in the hospital population.

Intra-abdominal hypertension is defined (arbitrarily) as a sustained intra-abdominal pressure of greater than 12mmHg and can be graded as shown in ● Table 3.3.

Table 3.3. Grading of intra-abdominal hypertension.	
Grade 1	12-15mmHg
Grade 2	16-20mmHg
Grade 3	21-25mmHg
Grade 4	>25mmHg

Abdominal compartment syndrome requires the new onset of organ dysfunction combined with either an intra-abdominal pressure of >20mmHg or an abdominal perfusion pressure (APP = MAP-IAP) of <50mmHg. (APP = abdominal perfusion pressure; IAP = intra-abdominal pressure; MAP = mean arterial pressure.)

2) What are the risk factors for developing IAH and abdominal compartment syndrome?

Risk factors

- Retroperitoneal expansion:
  - bleeding from a ruptured abdominal aortic aneurysm (AAA);
  - bleeding from a fractured pelvis;
  - pancreatitis.
- Liver transplant — one third of recipients had abdominal pressures >25mmHg in one study.
- Intra-abdominal pathology:
  - ascites;
  - bowel distension — from obstruction, malignancy or from excess bowel handling during intra-abdominal surgery;
  - reduction of large hernias;
  - closure of abdominal wall under tension.
- Sepsis — large-volume crystalloid replacement and leaky capillaries leading to third space fluid losses and tissue oedema.
- Burns — large-volume crystalloid replacement as for sepsis.
- Peritoneal dialysis.

3) How can intra-abdominal pressure be measured?

It should be noted that the intra-abdominal pressure varies within the respiratory cycle and with different patient positions. Serial measurements should be undertaken with the patient supine and at the end of expiration:

- Direct measurement. A pressure transducer can be introduced through the abdominal wall to directly measure pressure. This is infrequently used as it risks direct damage to structures within the abdomen.

101

- Indirect measurement. In all these methods the pressure within a hollow viscus is measured and it is assumed that the wall of this viscus is a transducer and therefore represents intra-abdominal pressure:
    - bladder — this is the most common method as it is the least invasive and patients who require their abdominal pressure to be measured invariably have a urinary catheter *in situ*. An electronic transducer can be integrated with the catheter or the height of a column of static fluid (manometry) in the drainage tube can be physically measured above the symphysis pubis (N.B. this gives a pressure in cmH_2O [or urine] rather than mmHg and requires sufficient urine volume);
    - intravenous catheter — a central venous line can be introduced into the femoral vein and directed into the inferior vena cava within the abdomen. The distal port of this central venous catheter (CVC) can be transduced as for central venous pressure and will give an accurate trend of IAP;
    - gastric — can be continuous or intermittent and involves inserting a gastric balloon catheter into the stomach and measuring the pressure in the balloon which has a known quantity of air within it;
    - colonic/uterine — a fluid-filled balloon catheter is introduced and transduced to give IAP.

4) What are the physiological consequences of abdominal compartment syndrome?

Cardiovascular

- Raised IAP causes a reduction in venous return from the lower extremities. This leads to venous stasis in the legs and an increased deep vein thrombosis risk as well as a reduction in cardiac preload and therefore a reduced cardiac output.

- Raised IAP causes splinting and elevation of the diaphragm — pressing upon the base of the heart and causing a direct reduction in contractility. Movement of the mediastinum may also cause disruption to venous inflow and further reduce preload.

Pulmonary

- Splinting and raising of the diaphragm leads to direct compression of lung tissue and a reduced functional residual capacity. Patients being mechanically ventilated will require higher ventilator pressures due to reduced compliance. This may lead to pulmonary barotrauma. The effects of all these factors will lead to atelectasis, increased shunt and reduced oxygen diffusion capacity in the lungs which may cause hypoxaemia.

Gastrointestinal

- The vascular supply of the gut mesentery is very susceptible to raised IAP — even at pressures of 10mmHg. The initial effect is to reduce venous drainage of the mesentery which in turn leads to oedema within the bowel and a further rise in intra-abdominal pressure. Eventually the pressure causes reduced arterial flow and bowel ischaemia.
- Hypoperfusion of the gut affects the patency of the mucosal barrier and allows translocation of bacteria into the systemic circulation leading to sepsis and multi-organ failure.

Renal

- Renal failure occurs as a result of:
  - reduced venous drainage of the glomerulus due to the direct effect of raised IAP;
  - reduced arterial perfusion as a result of a low cardiac output state — see the cardiovascular section above.
- Plasma levels of renin, angiotensin and aldosterone are elevated.

Neurological

- Similar to the transient elevation in intracranial pressure (ICP) observed during coughing, a prolonged rise in IAP causes a prolonged elevation in ICP.

Hepatic

- Synthetic function of the liver is reduced by a rise in IAP by as little as 10mmHg. Clinically, this may manifest as an inability or reduced ability to clear lactate.

5) What is the management of abdominal compartment syndrome?

General/supportive

The aim is to reduce the intra-abdominal contents and pressure. This can be achieved by:

- Nasogastric drainage.
- Bowel content elimination — enemas and laxatives.
- Drainage of ascites if present — with intravenous albumin replacement.
- Percutaneous drainage of intra-abdominal collections/abscesses.
- Adequate analgesia — this will allow for improved abdominal wall compliance and reduced muscle tone.
- Patient position — supine is the best position for reducing IAP but this must be balanced with respiratory function and the risk of aspiration and ventilator-associated pneumonia.

- Intubation and ventilation may be required for respiratory compromise.
- In ventilated patients:
  - adequate sedation to improve abdominal wall compliance;
  - consideration of muscle relaxation to obliterate the contribution of the abdominal wall musculature on IAP;
  - ventilator settings — it may be necessary to reduce tidal volumes or ventilator pressures and allow permissive hypercapnia. The use of PEEP needs to be considered — a higher PEEP may improve oxygenation (and allow for lower inspiratory pressures) but may also splint the diaphragm and contribute to IAP. A high PEEP may also further reduce the venous return and cardiac preload.
- Haemodynamics — fluid administration may temporarily improve venous return and therefore perfusion, but risks leaking from the vasculature and into abdominal tissues worsening IAP. Fluid alone cannot 'treat' abdominal compartment syndrome and there is no role for diuretics either.

Surgical

The only definitive management is surgical decompression — laparostomy — but there is no defined point at which it should be undertaken. Some surgeons advocate early decompression when IAH is present before abdominal compartment syndrome and multi-organ failure occurs. Others use organ perfusion pressures with a threshold perfusion pressure of 50mmHg as an indication for surgical decompression. Once the abdomen is open, pressures may reduce and organ perfusion is restored. The open abdomen needs to be managed with temporary closure and then delayed definitive closure. If this occurs prematurely, then abdominal compartment syndrome can recur.

Summary of Key Points

- Normal abdominal pressure is 5-7mmHg. Abdominal hypertension begins at >12mmHg.
- Risk factors include any increase in the volume of tissue or fluid within the abdomen — including high-volume fluid resuscitation in the critically ill with capillary leak.
- Intra-abdominal pressure can be measured directly or indirectly using pressure transducers.
- Raised intra-abdominal pressure affects almost all body systems both within and without the abdomen.
- Definitive treatment is surgical decompression but supportive measures may suffice.

References

1. Kirkpatrick AW, Roberts DJ, De Waele J, *et al*. Intra-abdominal hypertension and the abdominal compartment syndrome: updated consensus definitions and clinical practice guidelines from the World Society of the Abdominal Compartment Syndrome. *Intensive Care Med* 2013; 39: 1190.

2. Malbrain ML, Chiumello D, Pelosi P, *et al*. Incidence and prognosis of intraabdominal hypertension in a mixed population of critically ill patients: a multiple-center epidemiological study. *Crit Care Med* 2005; 33: 315.

3. Dries DJ. Abdominal compartment syndrome: toward less-invasive management. *Chest* 2011; 140: 1396.

SET 4

1) What are the colour codes and contents of fire extinguishers in the UK?

Fire extinguishers in the United Kingdom are all red in colour and have colour-coded bands to indicate their contents (● Table 4.1).

Table 4.1. Fire extinguishers and colour-coded bands.

Red band	Water, for use on wood, paper, textile and solid material fires
Black band	Carbon dioxide, for use on liquid and electrical fires
Cream band	Foam, for use on wood, paper, textile and liquid fires
Blue band	Dry powder, for use on wood, paper, textile, liquid and electrical fires
Yellow band	Wet chemical, for use on wood, paper, textile and cooking medium fires

2) How can we minimise the risk of fire breaking out on the intensive care unit?

Intensive care units are at an elevated risk of fire as a result of the use of open breathing circuits utilising high flows and fractions of oxygen. In order to mitigate against this risk there needs to be measures to ensure that there are no ignition sources or other sources of fuel. These measures include:

- Regular testing of electrical equipment to ensure faults and the potential for sparks do not occur.
- Prohibiting personal electronic equipment or charging devices that have not been tested to ensure safety — both for staff and patients.
- Safe use of compressed gas cylinders — placing them in proper holders rather than on patient beds, correct and judicious use of lubricants applied by the manufacturer.
- Regular removal of waste to prevent a build-up in clinical areas or corridors.
- Specified areas to store waste before it is removed from the clinical area.
- Regular cleaning of hard-to-reach areas to prevent the build-up of lint and flammable debris, e.g. within the ventilation system.

In addition to these measures, all new builds or refurbishments of critical care units need to conform to modern safety standards in terms of fireproof materials and fire doors.

3) How should intensive care units prepare themselves for evacuation if there is a fire?

Every intensive care unit should have a comprehensive fire plan which should be regularly rehearsed as a table top, single patient, whole unit and whole hospital exercise. The fire plan should form part of induction training for all new staff to a unit.

Each bed space should have a dedicated 'fire box' which contains a full oxygen cylinder, a self-inflating bag-valve-mask and instructions as to what to do in the event of a fire.

Upon the discovery of a fire or sounding of the alarm, there should be clear instructions from the nurse in charge pertaining to preparation and then activation of the evacuation plan with a clearly identified destination to set up a temporary critical care area — usually theatre recovery or a remote critical care area.

On activation of the alarm, and the decision to evacuate, each nurse should return to their bed space and do the following:

- Ask all ambulatory visitors to evacuate via the nearest fire escape.
- Stop all unnecessary infusions and feed.
- Transfer all other infusion pumps onto the bed.
- Put the patient monitor onto the bed — small box, if the system allows.
- Switch to the emergency oxygen and hand ventilation device in the fire box.
- Put patient notes on the bed.
- Ensure bed and ancillaries (mattress, etc.) are unplugged.
- Prepare for evacuation.

The nurse and consultant in charge should make the decision about switching off the piped oxygen supply and decide upon the order that patients are evacuated.

4) What safeguards are there in the intensive care unit to mitigate against power failure?

There are several levels of redundancy built into hospital power supplies to try and ensure that vital equipment does not suffer in the event of failure of one form of power provision.

The entire hospital is connected to the main power supply from the national grid. This provides a consistent supply of electricity to a hospital, but there is a risk of failure of this system.

The hospital has a secondary power supply which is provided by on-site generators. These start automatically if the voltage supply from the mains falls below 80% of normal for 2 seconds or more. There is a delay in the detection and start of this back-up system so there may be a loss of power to secondary power supply sockets of up to 15 seconds. Not all hospital sockets are on the secondary power supply — those designated sockets are red in colour. Only those systems which have internal battery back-up (such as monitors) and systems that can afford to temporarily lose power (such as surgical diathermy) should be plugged into these sockets — this ensures that there is no critical loss of function during changeover.

The tertiary back-up system is termed the 'uninterruptable power supply' and is formed from a bank of batteries which supply blue-coloured plugs. Equipment that cannot afford a loss of power for any time at all should be plugged into these sockets, e.g. renal replacement therapy machines. The duration that the uninterruptable power supply will function depends upon the size of the battery bank and the power load placed upon it.

Many systems have integral battery back-up systems, e.g. infusion pumps and monitors so that if there is a catastrophic failure of power across all back-up systems there will still be a period of functionality from the internal battery supply.

Intensive care units should have a comprehensive power failure plan which includes:

- Alternate light sources at each bed space and at the staff bases.
- Oxygen cylinders and a method of manually ventilating patients at each bed space in case of catastrophic failure and the loss of mechanical ventilators.
- Portable pulse oximeters and manual sphygmomanometers available to allow ongoing monitoring.
- Plans for movement of patients to alternative areas if the power supply is expected not to be restored within a short period of time.

Summary of Key Points

- Fire extinguishers in the UK have changed in the last few years and are now all red with different coloured stripes to indicate their contents pertinent to different types of fires.
- Fire is an unlikely event in the ICU but should be planned for and evacuation procedures practised regularly.
- There are four levels of power supply within a hospital: mains, secondary, uninterruptable and battery back-up.

References

1. Miles LF, Scheinkestel CD, Downey GO. Environmental emergencies in theatre and critical care areas: power failure, fire, and explosion. *Contin Educ Anaesth Crit Care Pain* 2015; 15(2): 78-83.

2. Kelly FE, Hardy R, Cook TM, *et al.* Managing the aftermath of a fire on intensive care caused by an oxygen cylinder. *J Intensive Care Soc* 2014; 15(4): 283.

Local anaesthetic systemic toxicity

1) What is local anaesthetic systemic toxicity (LAST)?

LAST

- Toxicity occurs when an overdose of local anaesthetic enters the systemic circulation, for example, due to an inadvertent intravenous injection.
- Maximum doses vary according to the drug, patient age and weight, vascularity of the site and individual tolerance. The toxic doses of commonly used local anaesthetics are listed in ● Table 4.2 below.
- The absorption is influenced by the vascularity of the site, which is presented below with the order listed from the most vascular and potentially lethal to the least:
  - intravenous;
  - intercostal;
  - caudal epidural;
  - lumbar epidural;
  - brachial plexus;
  - subcutaneous.

Table 4.2. Toxic doses of commonly used local anaesthetics.

Drug	Onset (min)	Duration (min)	Max dose (mg/kg)	Characteristics
Lidocaine	2 low pKa = rapid onset	15-60	3	Medium-acting amide Moderate vasodilatation Class 1b anti-arrhythmic
Lidocaine with adrenaline	2	120-360	7	Adrenaline provides local vasoconstriction reducing the absorption and breakdown of the lidocaine, thus extending its duration of action
Bupivacaine	5	180-240	2	Long-acting amide Racemic mixture of R and S enantiomers Prolonged cardiotoxicity
Levobupivacaine	5	180-240	2	S enantiomer Less toxic than bupivacaine as binds less strongly to myocardium Shorter motor block than bupivacaine
Prilocaine	2 low pKa = rapid onset	15-30	6	Medium-acting amide No vasodilation Rapid metabolism Low toxicity Metabolites cause methaemoglobinaemia

2) What risk factors are associated with LAST?

Procedural factors

- Accidental intravascular injection, reduced by regular aspiration.

Maximum safe dose exceeded

This can be as a result of the following factors:

- Fast injection with high dose of local anaesthetic.
- Delayed recognition of toxicity in anaesthetised or sedated patients.
- Infusions not carefully monitored or using incorrect pumps, settings or connections.

3) Briefly outline the pathophysiology of LAST.

Local anaesthetic toxicity presents with neurological and cardiovascular sequelae.

The proposed pathophysiology suggests that the local anaesthetic causes antagonism of oxidative phosphorylation in mitochondria. The heart and brain are both dependent upon aerobic metabolism rendering them both very vulnerable.

Another possible mechanism includes non-neuronal sodium channel inhibition. The theory is that blockage of inhibitory pathways within the cerebral cortex causes excitatory nerve activity. This manifests as tingling, agitation and seizures. In both cardiac and neuronal tissues, the initial excitability is followed by depression. This will result in myocardial negative inotropy, coma and cardiac arrest.

4) A) How can you recognise local anaesthetic toxicity clinically?

Prompt recognition is vital to avoid complications. Be aware that toxicity does not always occur immediately following an injection.

Mild toxicity

- Peri-oral tingling, lightheadedness, tinnitus, blurred vision.

Severe toxicity

- Neurological — sudden alteration in mental status, agitation, loss of consciousness, seizures, coma.
- Cardiovascular — sinus bradycardia, conduction deficit, asystole and ventricular tachyarrhythmias, ECG abnormalities include:
  - prolongation of QRS and PR interval;
  - AV block;
  - T-wave changes.

B) What investigations would you order and what might you see for someone suspected of having LAST?

- Severe toxicity is an emergency and requires immediate resuscitation.
- Initiation of therapy does not require laboratory confirmation.
- Consider taking blood for analysis but do not delay treatment.
- Investigations — arterial blood gas as part of resuscitation.

5) What are the management priorities?

General measures

- Stop the injection or infusion.
- This is a medical emergency and concurrent assessment, management and resuscitation should follow an 'airway, breathing, circulation, disability and exposure' approach.
- All cases of local anaesthetic toxicity should be reported to the National Patient Safety Agency (NPSA).

Medical pharmacological

- Treat convulsions with benzodiazipines — midazolam, lorazepam or diazepam. Consider induction of anaesthesia with propofol or thiopentone.
- Give an IV bolus of 20% lipid emulsion (e.g. Intralipid®), 1.5ml/kg over 1 minute.
- Start an infusion of lipid emulsion at 15ml/kg/hr.
- At 5 minutes repeat the bolus and double the infusion rate if there has been no response.
- A further bolus can be given if cardiovascular stability has not been restored after a further 5 minutes. The maximum recommended dose is 12ml/kg of 20% lipid emulsion within the first hour.
- If the patient suffers cardiac arrest, commence CPR and advanced life support (ALS), and manage as above; recovery may take greater than an hour and consider the use of cardiopulmonary bypass.

Summary of Key Points

- Prompt recognition and resuscitation are vital to avoid cardiovascular collapse.
- If cardiac arrest occurs, recovery may take greater than an hour and consider cardiopulmonary bypass.
- The route, drug chosen and patient factors, e.g. pregnancy, must be carefully considered to avoid accidental overdose.

References

1. Dewaele S, Santos A. NYSORA - The New York School of Regional Anesthesia. Toxicity of local anesthetics, 2017. Nysora.com. Available from: http://www.nysora.com/mobile/regional-anesthesia/foundations-of-ra/3075-toxicity-of-local-anesthetics.html.

2. Prout J, Jones T, Martin D. *Advanced Training in Anaesthesia*, 1st ed. Oxford University Press, 2014.

3. Allman K, Wilson I. *Oxford Handbook of Anaesthesia*, 2nd ed. Oxford University Press, 2016.

Antibiotics in critical care

1) List the mechanisms of antibacterial action and some antibiotic examples in each class.

Antibiotics are pharmacological agents that selectively kill or inhibit the growth of bacterial cells. Bacteriocidal antibiotics kill bacteria. Bacteriostatic antibiotics prevent further replication of bacteria and rely on an intact immune system to clear infection. Antibiotics can be divided into different classes according to their mechanism of action outlined below.

Inhibition of cell wall synthesis

ß-lactams
- Penicillins:
    - ß-lactamase-sensitive, e.g. benzylpenicillin, phenoxymethyl-penicillin (V);
    - ß-lactamase-resistant, e.g. flucloxacillin, methicillin;
    - extended spectrum:
        - aminopenicillins, e.g. amoxicillin, ampicillin;
        - carboxypenicillins, e.g. ticarcillin, carbenicillin;
        - ureidopenicillins, e.g. piperacillin.
- Cephalosporins:
    - 1st generation, e.g. cephalexin, cefadrine;
    - 2nd generation, e.g. cefuroxime, cefaclor;
    - 3rd generation, e.g. cefotaxime, ceftriaxone;
    - 4th generation, e.g. cefepime;
    - 5th generation, e.g. ceftobiprole.
- Carbapenems, e.g. ertapenem:
    - antipseudomonal, e.g. meropenem.
- Monobactams, e.g. aztreonam.
- ß-lactamase inhibitors, e.g. clavulanic acid.

Glycopeptide derivatives
Glycopeptide derivatives, e.g. vancomycin, teicoplanin.

Inhibition of protein synthesis

● Aminoglycosides, e.g. gentamicin, tobramycin, amikacin.
● Macrolides, e.g. erythromycin, clarithromycin, azithromycin.
● Tetracyclines, e.g. tetracycline, doxycycline.
● Lincosamides, e.g. clindamycin.
● Chloramphenicol.

Inhibition of bacterial nucleic acid synthesis

● Sulfonamides, e.g. sulfisoxazole.
● Pyrimidine derivatives, e.g. trimethoprim.
● Rifamycins, e.g. rifampicin.
● Quinolones, e.g. ciprofloxacin, levofloxacin, moxifloxacin.
● Metronidazole.

Others

● Cyclic lipopeptides, e.g. daptomycin.
● Glycylcyclines, e.g. tigecycline.
● Oxazolidinones, e.g. linezolid.
● Lipiarmycins, e.g. fidaxomicin.

2) Which factors contribute to the success or failure of antibiotic treatment?

● Resilience/vulnerability of the host.
● Virulence of the organism.
● Use of appropriate antibiotic therapy:
    - sensitivity;
    - tissue penetration.

- Rapid source control:
  - removal of foreign bodies, such as implantable devices and catheters, and devitalized tissue;
  - drainage of abscesses.

3) How do bacteria transfer the genetic material conferring resistance between themselves?

- Transformation — the introduction, uptake and expression of foreign DNA into a cell — such DNA is often described as "naked", i.e. is freely floating in whichever extracellular medium the bacteria currently occupy.
- Transduction — bacterial DNA is moved from one bacterium to another by a viral vector called a bacteriophage.
- Conjugation — the transfer of DNA in plasmid form from one bacterial cell to another when their cell walls come into contact.
- Transposons — a segment of DNA which moves locus from one genome to another but with parent to offspring transfer. Sometimes referred to as a "jumping gene", if the transposon picks up a piece of DNA which confers resistance, it can transfer this between bacteria.

4) A) Which factors contribute to antibiotic resistance?

- Increasing age.
- Illness severity.
- Prolonged ICU stay.
- Prior antibiotic usage.
- Exposure to indwelling devices, e.g. central venous catheters and tracheal tubes.
- Inappropriate antibiotic selection, e.g. prolonged courses of broad-spectrum antibiotics.
- Poor infection prevention, control and antibiotic stewardship.

B) Why is dealing with resistance important?

Antibiotic resistance poses a significant threat to public health. Despite increasing strains of resistant bacteria, there are a few new classes of antibiotic on the horizon. Infections due to resistant organisms are associated with:

- Higher mortality and morbidity.
- Longer ICU and hospital stays.
- Higher healthcare costs.

5) List some strains of bacteria increasingly recognised for their resistance.

The ESCAPE acronym is useful to remember (● Table 4.3).

Table 4.3. ESCAPE acronym.

Enterococcus faecium (vancomycin resistance — VRE).

Staphylococcus aureus (methicillin resistance — MRSA, vancomycin intermediate resistance — VISA, vancomycin resistance — VRSA).

Clostridium difficile.

Acinetobacter baumannii (carbapenem, cephalosporin, aminoglycoside and quinolone resistance).

Pseudomonas aeruginosa (carbapenem resistance).

Enterobacteriaceae (extended-spectrum ß-lactamase-producing organisms — ESBLs, encompassing *Klebsiella pneumoniae*, *Enterobacter* species and *Escherichia coli* — 3rd generation cephalosporin and carbapenem resistance).

6) What are the main principles of antibiotic stewardship?

- Leadership and multi-disciplinary teamwork including intensivists, microbiologists and pharmacists.
- Surveillance of local microflora and antibiotic resistance patterns.
- Admission resistance screening.
- Appropriate microscopy and culture sampling prior to commencing antibiotics.
- Evidence-based prescribing guidelines including:
  - empirical antibiotic dosing, route, duration;
  - prescription review after 48-72 hours, with cessation or de-escalation from broad-spectrum to narrower-spectrum antibiotics according to culture sensitivities;
  - conversion from parenteral to enteral antibiotics;
  - monitoring advice;
  - contingency plans for treatment failure.
- Antibiotic cycling to reduce selection pressure.
- Formulary restriction and persuasive interventions.
- Prospective audit and quality improvement.
- Revision and feedback.
- Educational resources and training to ensuring appropriate antibiotic use.
- Information technology and computer assistance support.

In summary, the aim is to eradicate infection whilst minimising complications: the right drug, at the right dose, at the right time, for the right duration (customized to the patient with the shortest duration to ensure effective treatment whilst avoiding resistance).

Summary of Key Points

- Antibiotics are pharmacological agents that selectively kill or inhibit the growth of bacterial cells. They can be classified according to their mechanism of action.
- Antibiotic resistance poses a significant threat to public health. Despite increasing strains of resistant bacteria (ESCAPE acronym), there are a few new classes of antibiotic on the horizon.
- Therefore, it is crucial to pay close attention to the principles of antibiotic stewardship.

References

1. Varley AJ, Williams H, Fletcher S. Antibiotic resistance in the intensive care unit. *Contin Educ Anaesth Crit Care Pain* 2009; 9(4): 114-8.
2. Johnson I, Banks V. Antibiotic stewardship in critical care. *BJA Education* 2017; 17(4): 111-6.

Cardiac output monitoring

1)   What is cardiac output?

Cardiac output is the volume of blood ejected from the left ventricle per minute. It is a product of stroke volume and heart rate. It is influenced by preload, afterload and contractility. The cardiac index is the cardiac output adjusted for body surface area.

2)   What is the mean arterial pressure (MAP?)

This is the average arterial blood pressure throughout the cardiac cycle. MAP is calculated as diastolic blood pressure + 1/3 (systolic — diastolic blood pressure).

3)   What clinical and biochemical indicators can be used to estimate cardiac output?

Clinical signs include:

- Mental state.
- Heart rate.
- Capillary refill time.
- Urine output.
- Temperature.
- Skin temperature, in particular core/peripheral temperature gradient.

Blood pressure is a poor indicator of cardiac output as catecholamine-mediated vasoconstriction can compensate for a low cardiac-output state to a certain degree.

Lactate is produced when cellular metabolism is anaerobic. It is metabolised to pyruvate and glucose in the liver and so is a marker both of tissue hypoxia and liver hypoperfusion. It can be used to monitor response to therapy.

4)   What is the Fick principle?

The Fick principle is based on blood flow to an organ being determined using a marker substance if the concentration of marker substance in arterial blood supplying the organ, and concentration of marker substance leaving a target organ, are known.

5)   What methods of cardiac output monitoring are you aware of, and how can you classify them?

Cardiac output monitors can be classified as non-invasive, minimally-invasive and invasive.

Non-invasive/minimally-invasive

Echocardiography
Focused echocardiography in intensive care is gaining increasing recognition as a rapid non-invasive method of estimating cardiac output, as well as a diagnostic tool to look for pericardial effusion, right ventricular dilatation, valvular function, regional motion wall abnormalities and left ventricular function. The disadvantages are that it is not continuous and is user-dependent. Transoesophageal echocardiography may be used, although this requires additional equipment, a skilled operator and serial measurements are difficult.

Transoesophageal Doppler

Transoesophageal Doppler measures blood flow in the descending aorta via an ultrasound probe sited in the mid to distal oesophagus. The Doppler equation is used to produce a continuous waveform and can be used to measure stroke volume, preload, afterload, contractility and vascular resistance. It can measure dynamic changes in cardiac output and is relatively quick and easy to use. Its model does assume aortic cross-section based on demographic information, and that 70% of total cardiac output passes through the descending aorta, which may not be the case in severe hypovolaemia.

Thoracic impedance

Electrical impedance of the thorax changes throughout the cardiac and respiratory cycles, as blood volume changes. The rate of change is dependent upon cardiac output. Absolute values are less important than trends, but this method is not well validated in critical illness.

Carbon dioxide measurement

Using the Fick principle, carbon dioxide production in a closed loop breathing circuit can be used to estimate blood delivery to the lung, and therefore cardiac output. Differences between ventilation and perfusion introduce inaccuracies to this method.

Uncalibrated pulse contour analysis

Using a proprietary algorithm, based on data obtained in healthy volunteers, the arterial waveform can be analysed in order to provide an estimation of stroke volume variation and cardiac output. It is less accurate than calibrated methods.

Invasive

Calibrated pulse contour analysis

Transpulmonary lithium or thermodilution can be used to calibrate a pulse contour analysis device. This provides more accurate results than uncalibrated methods, and can be used to derive additional data such as the global end-diastolic volume index and extravascular lung water indices. Lithium dilution does not require central venous access whereas thermodilution does.

Pulmonary artery catheterisation
A Swan-Ganz catheter can be floated into the pulmonary artery and used to measure pulmonary capillary wedge pressure, a surrogate of left atrial pressure. Thermistors on the catheter can also be used for thermodilution methods to measure cardiac output. Direct administration of drugs to the pulmonary circulation can also be achieved. It requires additional training to site the catheter, and may be complicated by pulmonary infarction, haemorrhage and pulmonary embolus. Large studies have failed to demonstrate a mortality benefit with their use and they have fallen out of favour recently outside of specialist centres.

Cardiac catheterisation
Cardiac catheterisation is not used in the critical care setting.

6) What are the normal values for the Global End-Diastolic Volume Index (GEDI), Intrathoracic Blood Volume Index (ITBI) and stroke volume variation (SVV)?

These measured values are all a measure of preload, and changes within them can be used to predict ongoing fluid responsiveness.

- GEDI — 680-800ml/m^2.
- ITBI — 850-1000ml/m^2.
- SVV — <10%.

Summary of Key Points

- Clinical, biochemical, non-invasive and invasive methods can be used to measure cardiac output.
- Blood pressure is a poor indicator of cardiac output.
- There are advantages and disadvantages to each method, but generally cardiac output should be measured in critically unwell patients who require volume resuscitation or vasopressor support, particularly in the initial stages of resuscitation.

References

1.   Thiele RH, Bartels K, Gan TJ. Cardiac output monitoring: a contemporary assessment and review. *Crit Care Med* 2015; 43(1): 177-85.

Management of raised intracranial pressure (ICP)

1) What contributes to intracranial pressure and what causes ICP to be raised?

Reported 'normal' intracranial pressure varies between 7 and 15mmHg in supine adults and is contributed to by the contents of the cranial vault including:

- Brain parenchyma — approximately 80%.
- Blood in both the venous and arterial system — approximately 10%.
- Cerebrospinal fluid (CSF) — approximately 10%.

The contents of the cranial vault create a fixed volume equilibrium (Monro-Kellie hypothesis).

Intracranial pressure is physiologically and transiently raised by coughing, straining or through Valsalva manoeuvres, which can lead to pressure rises of up to 50mmHg. A persistently elevated ICP >20-25mmHg has a significant impact, with reduced cerebral perfusion pressure (CPP) — this being equal to the difference between mean arterial pressure (MAP) and ICP.

Causes of an elevated intracranial pressure include:

- Mass lesions — tumours and abscesses.
- Haematomas — in various planes of meninges and brain tissue.
- Cerebral oedema following hypoxic insult, severe trauma or a cerebral infarction.
- Increased CSF production, e.g. from a choroid plexus papilloma.
- Decreased CSF absorption or blockage of CSF drainage, e.g. by blood debris following a subarachnoid haemorrhage.
- Obstructive hydrocephalus.
- Venous obstruction, e.g. venous sinus thrombosis.
- Idiopathic/benign intracranial hypertension.

2) List some symptoms and signs of raised ICP.

Signs and symptoms of raised ICP include:

- Headache.
- Back pain.
- Vomiting.
- Papilloedema.
- Ocular palsies.
- Pupillary dilatation.
- Altered consciousness and coma.
- Cushing's triad:
  - raised systolic blood pressure (with a widened pulse pressure);
  - bradycardia;
  - abnormal respiratory pattern.

3) How can ICP be measured?

There are several theoretical ways of measuring ICP which are not used in clinical practice. These include:

- Ocular sonography — to measure optic sheath diameter. This has been shown to correlate with raised ICP if the diameter is >6mm.
- Measurement of intra-ocular pressure — contradictory studies show this to be both a useful correlation with ICP and of no correlation at all.
- Tissue resonance analysis — ultrasound-based assessment of brain tissue movement in response to the arterial pulsation as it passes. The resonance pattern changes predictably in the brain according to ICP, although only one small trial has been conducted so far.

Direct measurement of ICP is used in clinical practice and can be achieved by the insertion of:

- An intraventricular catheter — placed either at a craniotomy or through a burr hole and allows both measurement of ICP and drainage of CSF.
- An intraparenchymal monitor — placed via a small incision in the scalp after which a hollow 'bolt' is screwed into the skull. A needle is inserted through this bolt to puncture the dura to allow the passage of a pressure transducer into the brain parenchyma itself.
- A subarachnoid monitor — a fluid response system is placed in the extradural space, the dura is then punctured to allow communication between the system fluid and CSF. It is rarely used as the fluid drainage system is liable to block.

4)　How is raised ICP managed on the ICU?

Raised ICP, or a suspected raised ICP when it is not being formally measured, should be treated as a time critical emergency and managed with the following measures.

General

- An 'airway, breathing, circulation, disability and exposure' approach.
- Elevation of the head of the bed to 30° to encourage venous drainage.
- Support of end-organ perfusion and oxygenation — this may include airway protection by intubation (conducted with sufficient analgesia, sedation and muscle relaxation to prevent a rise in ICP associated with laryngoscopy or coughing), blood pressure support with fluid/blood product therapy to normovolaemia plus inotropes/vasopressors as required to a cerebral perfusion pressure of 60mmHg.

- Normoxia, normocarbia.
- Control of fever — avoidance of hyperthermia by pharmacological (paracetamol) and non-pharmacological (cooling pads/blankets/intravascular device) methods.
- Avoidance of circumferential tube ties/C-spine collars to reduce venous congestion and promote drainage. Traditionally, also the avoidance of internal jugular central lines for the same reason — although the risk associated with this may be mitigated by the need to increase cerebral perfusion pressure with vasoactive drugs via a central venous line.

Medical

- Osmotic therapy — use of mannitol (an osmotic diuretic) or hypertonic saline to reduce the water content of brain tissue by dehydrating the brain parenchyma. Mannitol causes a diuresis above that of hypertonic saline so this may have implications for circulating volume and therefore perfusion. Hypertonic saline has been shown to be more effective at reducing ICP than mannitol (and in a smoother profile) with a meta-analysis of the current trial data; however, clinical outcomes were not measured so debate remains as to which to use.
- Sedation — adequately sedated patients have a lower cerebral metabolic rate and therefore a lower oxygen demand, which is more easily met by a reduced supply. It also enables better ventilator synchronisation and avoids spikes in ICP due to high intrathoracic pressures and venous congestion.
- Control of seizures/suspected seizures — which increase cerebral oxygen demand and raise body temperature as well as directly increasing ICP.

5) What is the role of a decompressive craniectomy in the management of raised ICP?

The use of decompressive craniectomy has been shown to reduce intracranial pressure by as much as 70% if the dura is opened at the same time. However, its use has remained controversial and has been studied for different clinical indications. The most recent evidence suggests that in traumatic brain injury, decompressive craniectomy reduces mortality but increases the risk of long-term severe disability in the increased number of survivors. However, its use may still be indicated following malignant middle cerebral artery ischaemic stroke. Increasingly, the decision to undertake a decompressive craniectomy needs to be made on a case-by-case basis by senior neurosurgical and neurocritical care consultants.

Summary of Key Points

- Raised intracranial pressure occurs as a result of the expansion of any of the intracranial contents within the rigid confines of the skull vault.
- If raised intracranial pressure is suspected, investigation and monitoring should be instigated.
- Intracranial pressure can be monitored directly or inferred indirectly.
- Medical management and neuro parameters need to be strictly observed and manipulated to avoid loss of cerebral perfusion and oxygenation which will have a detrimental effect.
- Decompressive craniectomy may still be appropriate in specific circumstances but should be discussed on a case-by-case basis by senior clinicians.

References

1.   Soldatos T, Karakitsos D, Chatzimichail K, *et al*. Optic nerve sonography in the diagnostic evaluation of adult brain injury. *Crit Care* 2008; 12: R67.

2.   Lashutka MK, Chandra A, Murray HN, *et al*. The relationship of intraocular pressure to intracranial pressure. *Ann Emerg Med* 2004; 43: 585.

3.   Han Y, McCulley TJ, Horton JC. No correlation between intraocular pressure and intracranial pressure. *Ann Neurol* 2008; 64: 221.

4.   Michaeli D, Rappaport ZH. Tissue resonance analysis; a novel method for noninvasive monitoring of intracranial pressure. Technical note. *J Neurosurg* 2002; 96: 1132.

5.   Kamel H, Navi BB, Nakagawa K, *et al*. Hypertonic saline versus mannitol for the treatment of elevated intracranial pressure: a meta-analysis of randomized clinical trials. *Crit Care Med* 2011; 39: 554.

6.   Jourdan C, Convert J, Mottolese C, *et al*. Evaluation of the clinical benefit of decompression hemicraniectomy in intracranial hypertension not controlled by medical treatment. *Neurochirurgie* 1993; 39: 304.

7.   Hutchinson PJ, Kolias AG, Timofeev IS, RESCUEicp Trial Collaborators, *et al*. Trial of decompressive craniectomy for traumatic intracranial hypertension. RESCUEicp Trial. *N Engl J Med* 2016; 375(12): 1119-30.

Delirium

1) A) Define 'delirium'.

- Delirium is an acute confusional state characterised by fluctuating mental status, inattention, and either disorganised thinking or an altered level of consciousness. It can by hyperactive (agitated), hypoactive (inattentive, stuporous, withdrawn), or mixed.

B) Explain how widespread a problem delirium is amongst hospital inpatients.

- It is the commonest neuropsychiatric condition in hospital and is particularly prevalent in critical care, affecting up to 70% of ICU patients and 80% with APACHE scores >25.
- Delirium is grossly underdiagnosed (particularly hypoactive delirium) and is associated with:
  - increased duration of ventilation;
  - increased reintubation rate;
  - increased ICU and hospital length of stay;
  - long-term neurocognitive dysfunction;
  - increased healthcare costs;
  - increased mortality; delirious patients are 2-3 times more likely to die.

2) What are the common predisposing factors for delirium?

- Patient demographics:
  - age ≥65;
  - male sex.

- Cognitive status:
  - dementia;
  - cognitive impairment;
  - history of delirium;
  - depression.
- Functional status:
  - functional dependence;
  - immobility;
  - history of falls.
- Sensory impairment:
  - visual impairment;
  - hearing impairment.
- Dehydration and malnutrition.
- Alcohol abuse.
- Comorbidities:
  - severe illness;
  - chronic renal or hepatic disease;
  - history of CVA or other neurological disease;
  - trauma;
  - terminal illness;
  - HIV infection.

3) What are the common precipitating causes of delirium?

- Deliriogenic drugs:
  - opioids;
  - antidepressants;
  - anticonvulsants;
  - antihistamines;
  - antiemetics;
  - benzodiazepines;
  - corticosteroids;
  - diuretics;

- cardiovascular agents such as: atenolol, digoxin, dopamine, lidocaine.
- Metabolic, biochemical, hypoxic and haemodynamic derangement.
- Pain.
- Infection.
- Sleep deprivation — combination of environmental factors (noise, light, etc.) and critical illness.

4) Outline the Confusion Assessment Method for ICU (CAM-ICU) screening tool questions.

The CAM-ICU screening tool has a sensitivity of 81% and a specificity of 96% for the detection of delirium. It can be used for intubated patients.

- Acute change or fluctuating course of mental status:
  - is there an acute change from mental status baseline or has the patient's mental status fluctuated during the past 24 hours?
  - no = no delirium.
- Inattention:
  - the patient is instructed to "squeeze my hand when I say the letter 'A'";
  - SAVEAHAART or CASABLANCA is spelled out slowly by the person undertaking the CAM-ICU;
  - 0-2 errors = no delirium;
  - >2 errors, proceed.
- Altered level of consciousness:
  - Richmond Agitation Sedation Scale (RASS) other than zero = delirium present;
  - RASS zero, proceed.
- Disorganised thinking:
  - will a stone float on water?
  - are there fish in the sea?

- does one pound weigh more than two?
- do you use a hammer to hit a nail?
- ask the patient to "raise two fingers with one hand" and "do the same with the other hand";
- >1 error = delirium present.

5) What are the key prevention and management strategies for ICU delirium?

Non-pharmacological

- Promote continuity of nursing care.
- Optimise communication with visual and hearing aids.
- Provide appropriate cognitive stimulation and activity.
- Reorientate the patient verbally and visually, e.g. time and date clock.
- Identify and treat the precipitating cause, e.g. infection, pain.
- Sedation targets (RASS 0 or -1) and daily sedation holds.
- Encourage normal sleep pattern, e.g. dark and quiet at night.
- Early mobilisation.
- Avoid physical restraints.
- Avoid constipation.
- If distressed, try verbal de-escalation techniques.

Pharmacological

- Firstline: haloperidol.
- Atypical antipsychotics, e.g. olanzapine.
- Reserve benzodiazepines for patient or staff safety, or alcohol withdrawal.

Summary of Key Points

- Delirium is an acute confusional state characterised by fluctuating mental status, inattention, and either disorganised thinking or an altered level of consciousness.
- It is common, particularly in the ICU, but is often underdiagnosed with significant morbidity and mortality as a result.
- It is crucial to identify, and eliminate if possible, any precipitating causes.
- Use non-pharmacological and pharmacological means to prevent and manage ICU delirium.

References

1.   http://www.icudelirium.co.uk/.
2.   Alce TM, Page V, Vizcaychipi MP. Delirium uncovered. *J Intensive Care Soc* 2013; 14(1): 53-9.

SET5

1) What is the difference between Stevens-Johnson syndrome (SJS) and toxic epidermal necrolysis (TEN)?

SJS and TEN are conditions along the same spectrum of disease. These are rare, acute and potentially fatal conditions, related to a destructive cutaneous disease process. The skin lesions feature macules, erythema and blisters progressing to sheets of skin becoming detached, exposing dermis. SJS is at the less severe end of the spectrum, whilst TEN is severe and life-threatening. They are classified as severe cutaneous adverse reactions, the most common precipitant cause being drugs.

SJS

- Is generally less severe and usually only affects <10% of the body surface area.
- Affects mucous membranes usually in two or more sites — oral, genital and ocular.

TEN

- More severe and affects >30% of the body surface area.
- 90% have mucous membrane involvement.

2) What is the aetiology of SJS and TEN?

Causes of SJS/TEN include:

- Infective and inflammatory:
  - viral — patients with HIV infection are 100 times more likely to develop SJS/TEN, although the mechanism behind this is not fully understood but may be related to the range of medications they take;
  - bacterial — *Mycoplasma pneumoniae* is the second most common trigger for SJS/TEN.
- Autoimmune — patients with systemic lupus erythematosus (SLE) are at an increased risk of SJS/TEN, although SJS/TEN may have some crossover with severe cutaneous forms of SLE.
- Iatrogenic — drugs are the most common cause of SJS/TEN, usually occurring within the first 8 weeks of treatment. The most common causative agents are:
  - allopurinol;
  - lamotrigine;
  - sulfonamides;
  - nevirapine;
  - carbamazepine;
  - phenobarbitol.
- Neoplastic — malignancy of any sort may increase the risk of SJS/TEN but the causation may be due to the increased number of medications taken by people with cancers, with this being the underlying cause.
- Congenital genetic predispositions include:
  - HLA B15:02;
  - polymorphisms in genes encoding cytochrome p450 enzymes — which may expand the list of potentially causative medications.

3) What complications arise as a result of skin failure from any cause?

Patients with skin failure present a complex set of issues to the intensive care unit:

- Massive initial and ongoing fluid loss — especially in the burns patient where the fluid loss is exacerbated by the thermal injury. Fluid replacement calculations such as the Parkland formula should be undertaken for maintenance fluids and to replace losses. The skin should be dressed in such a way as to limit ongoing fluid losses. Inadequately treated, this can lead to organ hypoperfusion and the risk of acute kidney injury.
- Electrolyte imbalances as a result of the fluid losses and replacement — levels need to be carefully monitored and replaced.
- Superadded bacterial infections — due to the loss of the protective skin barrier but also as a result of the inflammatory response which promotes the translocation of bacteria across the bowel wall. The most common organisms are *Staphylococcus aureus* and *Pseudomonas*. Such infections should be aggressively treated but the role of prophylactic antibiotics remains controversial.
- Hypermetabolic state — correlates with an increased area of skin failure, especially in burns, with massive protein and lipid catabolism. Early nutritional support is essential in these cases.
- Hypothermia — an inability to thermoregulate effectively. Burns patients need to be in a temperature-controlled environment and can get cold very easily, e.g. when transferring to an operating theatre for debridement or skin grafting.

4) Outline the organisation of the Burn Care Network within the United Kingdom.

In England and Wales, burns services operate in a three-tiered system depending upon the severity and complexity of the burn indicating the level of input required:

- Burn facilities provide care for the least complex burns and are essentially at hospitals which have plastic surgery services but no specialised burn capability.
- Burn units care for patients with burns of a moderate size or severity and have access to specialised high dependency burns care.
- Burn centres provide the highest level of care with specialist burn intensive care units. They can care for complex burns. They also have access to other specialist facilities, so can manage patients who have other injuries/conditions.

5) Which patients should be discussed with a burn centre?

The following may benefit from care in a specialist burn unit or burn centre:

- All patients under 1 year, all patients under 2 years with >5% total body surface area (TBSA) burns, and elderly patients with significant comorbidities that could complicate management.
- Patients with burns >10% TBSA.
- Full-thickness burns.
- Burns to special areas (face, hands, feet, perineum, major joints).
- Burns plus an inhalational injury.
- Circumferential burns.
- Burns plus concomitant trauma — ideally a burn facility within a major trauma centre.
- Electrical burns including lightning strikes.
- Chemical burns.

Summary of Key Points

- SJS and TEN are disorders along the same spectrum, with TEN being more severe.
- The most common cause of SJS/TEN is medication.
- Skin failure is complex and there is a series of complications which need to be mitigated against.
- Burns services in the UK are made up of (from lowest acuity to highest acuity care) burn facilities, burn units and burn centres.
- Complex burns, for whatever reason, should be referred up the chain of burn care.

References

1. Mittmann N, Knowles SR, Koo M, *et al.* Incidence of toxic epidermal necrolysis and Stevens-Johnson syndrome in an HIV cohort: an observational, retrospective case series study. *Am J Clin Dermatol* 2012; 13: 49.

2. Ferrandiz-Pulido C, Garcia-Patos V. A review of causes of Stevens-Johnson syndrome and toxic epidermal necrolysis in children. *Arch Dis Child* 2013; 98: 998.

3. Ziemer M, Kardaun SH, Liss Y, Mockenhaupt M. Stevens-Johnson syndrome and toxic epidermal necrolysis in patients with lupus erythematosus: a descriptive study of 17 cases from a national registry and review of the literature. *Br J Dermatol* 2012; 166: 575.

4. Sassolas B, Haddad C, Mockenhaupt M, *et al.* ALDEN, an algorithm for assessment of drug causality in Stevens-Johnson syndrome and toxic epidermal necrolysis: comparison with case-control analysis. *Clin Pharmacol Ther* 2010; 88: 60.

5. Gravante G, Delogu D, Marianetti M, *et al.* Toxic epidermal necrolysis and Steven-Johnson syndrome in oncologic patients. *Eur Rev Med Pharmacol Sci* 2007; 11: 269.

Sodium disorders

1) Briefly describe sodium homeostasis.

Normal serum sodium is controlled between 134-146mmol/L. Sodium is the most abundant cation in the extracellular fluid (ECF) and consequently the major determinant of blood osmolality (number of osmoles per kilogram of solvent, independent of temperature and pressure, whereas osmolarity is the number of osmoles of solute per litre of solution).

Osmolality = $2(Na^+ + K^+)$ + glucose + urea (electrolytes in mmol/L)

Normal serum osmolality is 280-295mOsm/kg

Homeostasis is maintained by the hypothalamus (via osmoreceptors) and the renin angiotensin system (RAS) which compensates for changes in dietary sodium by altering renal absorption. Increases in ECF osmolality cause vasopressin (antidiuretic hormone, ADH) release which acts at the distal nephron to increase water reabsorption. It is important to note that increased fluid intake is guided by thirst which is possible only in conscious patients. Hypovolaemia stimulates renin release which via the RAS increases aldosterone release from the adrenal cortex. Reduced plasma sodium also increases aldosterone which acts on the collecting ducts to increase sodium and consequently water reabsorption. Atrial natriuretic peptide (ANP) aids fluid volume control. Key to homeostasis is the ability of the kidney to produce both highly concentrated and highly dilute urine, hence osmolality ranges from 50 to 1400mOsm/kg.

2) Define and classify disorders of low sodium.

Hyponatraemia is a serum sodium <135mmol/L and can be classified as mild (130-135mmol/L), moderate (125-129mmol/L) and severe (≤125mmol/L).

Hyponatraemia has many causes and can be broadly classified according to the volume status of the patient (● Table 5.1); it usually represents a relative excess of water. Sodium disorders and the treatment can be life-threatening if the altered plasma osmolality and consequent osmotic gradients are not understood.

Table 5.1. Causes of hyponatraemia.

Hypovolaemic	Normovolaemic	Hypervolaemic
Cerebral salt wasting syndrome (CSWS)	Syndrome of inappropriate ADH (SIADH)	SIADH
Diuretic therapy	Thiazide diuretics	Congestive cardiac failure
Diarrhoea & vomiting	Adrenal insufficiency	Nephrotic syndrome
Sweating	Hypothyroidism	Cirrhosis (vasodilatation causes release of vasoconstrictors including ADH)
Adrenal insufficiency	Iatrogenic	Renal failure
Blood loss		Iatrogenic (excessive fluid administration)
		'TURP' syndrome (fluid used to irrigate during transurethral resection of the prostate is absorbed by the vascular bed, 1.5L on average)

3) A) What is SIADH?

Hyponatraemia and hypo-osmolality resulting from inappropriately continued action of antidiuretic hormone (arginine vasopressin) leads to impaired excretion of water.

B) What are the possible causes of SIADH?

- Vascular:
  - CNS ischaemia and haemorrhage.
- Infective and inflammatory:
  - viral — HIV/AIDS;
  - bacterial — pneumonia;
  - asthma.
- Traumatic:
  - brain injury;
  - major surgery can also lead to increased secretion of ADH possibly pain-mediated.
- Iatrogenic and idiopathic:
  - drugs commonly implicated include thiazide diuretics, vincristine and cyclophosphamide;
  - rarer drug causes include haloperidol, selective serotonin reuptake inhibitors (SSRIs) and sodium valproate.
- Neoplastic:
  - commonly of the lung (particularly small cell carcinoma);
  - brain tumours.
- Congenital:
  - SIADH due to a V2 receptor gene mutation leading to excess water reabsorption.

4) Compare the diagnosis and treatment of SIADH and CSWS.

Neither condition has a diagnostic test. CSWS is a rare endocrine condition causing hyponatraemia and fluid depletion, and can occur secondary to tumours within and trauma to the brain. The otherwise normally functioning kidney excretes excessive sodium. The patient will produce large volumes of urine and if conscious will have excess thirst and salt craving.

Schwartz-Bartter criteria for SIADH

- Hyponatremia with corresponding hypo-osmolality.
- Continued renal excretion of sodium.
- Urine less than maximally dilute.
- Absence of clinical evidence of volume depletion.
- Absence of other causes of hyponatraemia.
- Correction of hyponatraemia by fluid restriction.

Patients with SIADH are euvolaemic or hypervolaemic and the hyponatraemia tends to improve with fluid restriction as it is due to a relative excess of water. CSWS causes hypovolaemia and hyponatraemia which will not improve with fluid restriction.

SIADH treatment

- Treat the cause.
- Mild/asymptomatic — water restriction.
- Acute moderate/severe hyponatraemia particularly with symptoms (seizures, coma) — correct sodium with hypertonic saline, loop diuretics, vasopressin 2 receptor antagonists. Note that treatment must be balanced against the risk of central pontine myelinolysis, particularly if chronic. Aim for 0.5-1mmol/L per hour and no more than a 10-12mmol/L rise in the first 24 hours.

5) Define hypernatraemia and list some common causes.

Hypernatraemia is a serum sodium >145mmol/L; it is less common than hyponatraemia and is most commonly due to dehydration. It can also occur following brain injury due to diabetes insipidus (DI) in which the reduced secretion of ADH causes a diuresis. Nephrogenic DI occurs when the kidney does not respond to ADH. Note that rapid correction of hypernatraemia can cause cerebral oedema.

Summary of Key Points

- Hypernatraemia and hyponatraemia can both be fatal; however, poor management can also increase morbidity and mortality.
- Formal diagnosis may be delayed due to a lack of specific diagnostic testing. Close monitoring and an awareness of the potential differentials are vital to ensure good patient care.
- Electrolyte disturbances can be caused by underlying endocrine pathology. This remains poorly understood; if in doubt consult expert help.

References

1. Hirst C, Allahabadia A, Cosgrove J. The adult patient with hyponatraemia. *BJA Education* 2014; 15(5): 248-52.

2. Cole C, Gottfried O, Liu J, Couldwell W. Hyponatremia in the neurosurgical patient: diagnosis and management. *Neurosurgical Focus* 2004; 16(4): 1-10.

3. Prout J, Jones T, Martin D. *Advanced Training in Anaesthesia*, 1st ed. Oxford University Press, 2014.

4. Bartter F, Schwartz W. The syndrome of inappropriate secretion of antidiuretic hormone. *Am J Med* 1967; 42(5): 790-806.

Respiratory extracorporeal membrane oxygenation (ECMO)

1) List the various indications for respiratory ECMO referral.

The most common indication for ECMO referral is refractory respiratory failure despite conventional lung-protective ventilation. This may be as a result of:

- Pneumonia.
- Acute respiratory distress syndrome (ARDS).
- Acute graft versus host disease.
- Pulmonary contusion.
- Smoke inhalation.
- Status asthmaticus.
- Airway obstruction.
- Aspiration.
- Drowning.

ECMO may also be used as a bridge to lung transplantation.

2) A) What are the Berlin criteria for ARDS?

- Timing — within 1 week of a known clinical insult or new or worsening respiratory symptoms.
- Chest imaging — bilateral opacities — not fully explained by effusions, lobar/lung collapse, or nodules.
- Origin of oedema — respiratory failure not fully explained by cardiac failure or fluid overload, requires objective assessment, e.g. echocardiography to exclude hydrostatic oedema if there is no risk factor present.
- Oxygenation — categorised into mild/moderate/severe according to the PaO_2:FiO_2 ratio and PEEP.

151

B) What are the criteria for referral of patients with severe acute respiratory failure for consideration of retrieval and ECMO in the UK?

- Potentially reversible aetiology.
- Adequate gas exchange but an inability to achieve lung-protective ventilation:
  - tidal volumes >6ml/kg;
  - plateau pressure >30cmH$_2$O.
- Refractory respiratory failure despite lung-protective ventilation:
  - hypoxaemia (PaO$_2$:FiO$_2$ ratio <13.3kPa);
  - hypercapnia (at a level to cause a pH of <7.2).
- Severe asthma (pH <7.2).
- Murray score of 3 or more.
- Bronchopleural fistula.
- Seven days or less of FiO$_2$ >0.8, plateau pressure >30cmH$_2$O.

C) Which factors constitute the Murray score?

- PaO$_2$:FiO$_2$ ratio (kPa).
- Number of quadrants with infiltration seen on CXR (0-4).
- PEEP value on ventilator in cmH$_2$O.
- Compliance = tidal volume/(peak inspiratory pressure-PEEP) in ml/cmH$_2$O.

Each factor is scored between 0 and 4. These are then added together and divided by 4. A score of ≥2.5 constitutes severe lung injury and ECMO should be considered.

3) What is the rationale for respiratory ECMO?

- For appropriately selected patients with respiratory failure refractory to conventional approaches, ECMO provides a mechanism for achieving improved gas exchange whilst allowing appropriate lung-protective mechanical ventilation to rest the lungs and minimise secondary lung injury (ventilator-induced lung injury, VILI).

- Typically, optimal protective ventilation is achieved for patients on ECMO, with plateau pressures <25cmH$_2$O and reduced driving pressures.
- Cohorting patients in centres with a high volume of severe respiratory failure cases also improves their quality of care and outcomes.
- When a patient has been accepted, a team can be sent to retrieve the patient, sometimes placing the patient on ECMO at the local unit and transferring with mobile ECMO back to the severe respiratory failure centre.

4) A) What constitutes a venovenous ECMO (VV-ECMO) circuit?

- ECMO uses technology derived from modified cardiopulmonary bypass to allow gas exchange outside the patient's body.
- In VV-ECMO, venous blood is removed from the patient via a wide-bore cannula, a centrifugal pump drives the blood through a membrane facilitating gas exchange (oxygenation and carbon dioxide removal) and returns the blood to the patient's venous circulation via a warmer. Cannulation can be with a single-site dual-lumen catheter, or single/split-site separate catheters.

B) What are the common complications of respiratory ECMO?

- The extracorporeal circuit is thrombogenic so patients are routinely systemically anticoagulated.
- As a result, 50% of patients will suffer a haemorrhagic complication, intracranial haemorrhage being the most devastating.

- Infective complications are also common, related to indwelling lines, access sites and primary pathology.

5) What is the evidence base for severe respiratory failure centres and retrieval for ECMO in the UK?

- The CESAR trial randomised 180 adult patients with reversible respiratory failure for consideration for ECMO at Leicester (although not all received ECMO) versus conventional treatment. Survival at 6 months was 63% versus 47%.
- A further study matched 75 patients with suspected or confirmed H1N1 influenza referred to one of the four UK ECMO centres with non-ECMO-referred patients in a longitudinal cohort study during the 2009 epidemic. Hospital mortality was 23.7% versus 52.5% with individual matching.

Summary of Key Points

- A venovenous ECMO circuit consists of wide-bore venous cannulae, a centrifugal pump, a membrane oxygenator, and a heater.
- In principle, respiratory ECMO facilitates lung-protective ventilation whilst maintaining gas exchange.
- Despite potential complications, ECMO provides a survival benefit for selected patients with refractory respiratory failure of reversible aetiology.

References

1. Martinex G, Vuylsteke A. Extracorporeal membrane oxygenation in adults. *Contin Educ Anaesth Crit Care Pain* 2012; 12(2): 57-61.

2. Peek GJ, Mugford M, Tiruvoipati R. Efficacy and economic assessment of conventional ventilator support versus extracorporeal membrane oxygenation for severe adult respiratory failure (CESAR): a multicentre randomised controlled trial. *Lancet* 2009; 374: 1351-63.

3. Noah MA, Peek GJ, Finney SJ, *et al*. Referral to an extracorporeal membrane oxygenation center and mortality among patients with severe 2009 influenza A (H1N1). *JAMA* 2011; 306(15): 1659-68.

Sepsis

1) What is sepsis?

The Sepsis-3 group revised the definition of sepsis in 2016. Sepsis is defined as life-threatening organ dysfunction caused by a dysregulated host response to infection. Septic shock is defined as a subset of sepsis in which underlying circulatory and cellular metabolism abnormalities are profound enough to substantially increase mortality.

2) Can you tell me about the Sequential Organ Failure Assessment (SOFA) score?

The SOFA score is used to classify the degree of organ dysfunction in critical care patients, with a higher score increasing the probability of mortality (● Table 5.2). It is a combination of physiological and biochemical variables, looking at the PaO_2/FiO_2 ratio, platelet count, bilirubin concentration, mean arterial pressure/catecholamine requirements, GCS, serum creatinine and urine output. A SOFA score of 2 or greater carries an overall mortality of 10%.

The Sepsis-3 group recommended the use of the qSOFA (quick SOFA) score for septic shock screening outside of the critical care setting, as it does not require laboratory measurements, and a score of 2 or more should prompt further investigation for organ dysfunction.

qSOFA criteria:

- Respiratory rate >21/min.
- Altered mentation.
- Systolic blood pressure <100mmHg.

Table 5.2. SOFA score.

SOFA score	0	1	2	3	4
Respiratory PaO$_2$/FiO$_2$ ratio (kPa)	>53.3	<53.3	<40	<26.7 with respiratory support	<13.3 with respiratory support
Haematological Platelets x 10^3/μL	>150	<150	<100	<50	<20
Liver Bilirubin (μmol/L)	<20	20-32	33-101	102-204	>204
Cardiovascular Blood pressure	MAP >70mmHg	MAP <70mmHg	On dobutamine (any dose) or dopamine ≤5μg/kg/min	Noradrenaline or adrenaline <0.1μg/kg/min	Noradrenaline or adrenaline >0.1μg/kg/min
Neurological GCS	15	13-14	10-12	6-9	<6
Renal Creatinine (μmol/L)	<110	110-170	171-299	300-440	>440
Urine output	-	-	-	<500ml in 24 hours	<200ml in 24 hours

3) What are the key management points from the Surviving Sepsis Campaign?

The 2016 revision of the International Guidelines for the Management of Septic Shock (Surviving Sepsis Campaign) includes several recommendations. Of note, the use of protocolised early goal-directed therapy has been abandoned, as evidence from the PROCESS, PROMISE and ARISE trials failed to demonstrate a mortality benefit over usual care.

Key recommendations

Infection
- Administer broad-spectrum intravenous antimicrobial agents within 1 hour of sepsis recognition.
- Daily assessment for de-escalation of antimicrobials and narrowing spectrum of therapy based on culture results and clinical course.
- Obtain source control rapidly.

Resuscitation
- Administer 30ml/kg of crystalloid within 3 hours of recognition of tissue hypoperfusion, with further fluid administration based on using dynamic variables to assess fluid-responsiveness (e.g. pulse pressure variation).
- Noradrenaline should be the first-line vasopressor.
- In patients requiring vasopressor support, target a MAP of 65mmHg.

Mechanical ventilation
- In patients with septic shock and ARDS, target 6ml/kg predicted body weight tidal volume, with a plateau pressure of <30cmH$_2$O.

Governance
- Education and implementation of programs to improve sepsis care and screening.

4)   Can you describe some problematic bacterial infections that you may encounter in critical care?

Methicillin-resistant *Staphylococcus aureus* (MRSA) may be hospital-acquired or community-acquired. It is problematic as it is resistant to flucloxacillin, the usual first-line anti-staphylococcal agent, as well as other beta-lactam antibiotics, including cephalosporins. It is a Gram-positive aerobic organism that appears in clusters. The mecA gene is present in MRSA but not methicillin-sensitive *Staphylococcus aureus* (MSSA) and confers beta-lactam resistance. First-line therapy is usually a glycol peptide such as vancomycin or teicoplanin, although resistance to these antibiotics has been described. Linezolid is used as a second-line agent. Tigecycline and daptomycin may be used if linezolid fails. Ceftaroline, a novel 5th-generation cephalosporin, may also be effective in treating MRSA.

Panton-Valentine leukocydin (PVL) *Staphylococcus aureus* describes a species of *Staphylococcus aureus* that produce PVL, a toxin that destroys leucocytes. It is generally community-acquired and infection can occur in young, otherwise healthy individuals. Symptoms include recurrent skin infections/abscesses that do not improve despite antimicrobial treatment. Septicaemia, osteomyelitis and necrotising pneumonia may also be caused by PVL *Staphylococcus aureus*. PVL *Staphylococcus aureus* may be methicillin-sensitive or methicillin-resistant. First-line treatment for PVL pneumonia is linezolid with clindamycin. If there are features of severe disease, adding in rifampicin and IVIg is recommended. In osteomyelitis, teicoplanin or vancomycin with either gentamicin or rifampicin or sodium fusidate, are first-line agents. Second-line agents include linezolid, daptomycin and tigecycline.

Extended-spectrum beta-lactamase (ESBL) producing *Escherichia coli* are multi-antimicrobial-resistant organisms that may complicate ICU admission. The urinary tract is a common source, but they may be found in peritoneal fluid/collections, or the respiratory tract of hospitalised patients. They are resistant to beta-lactam antibiotics, quinolones, trimethoprim and tetracyclines. Carbapenems are frequently used as first-line agents. Colistin is used for treatment failure, but its nephrotoxicity limits its use.

Carbapenem-resistant enterobacteriaceae (CRE) produce carbapenemase and are frequently resistant to multiple other classes of antimicrobial agent. *E. coli*, *Enterobacter* and *Klebsiella* species are the usual culprits. Fosfomycin, gentamicin, tigecycline and colistin are all used in the treatment of CRE infection. Novel carbapenemase inhibitors are in development and may be deployed against CRE in the future.

Vancomycin-resistant enterococci (VRE) may cause infections of indwelling catheters, including urinary catheters and central venous catheters, as well as pneumonia and endocarditis. Nitrofurantoin, linezolid, daptomycin and tigecycline are generally effective, although daptomycin resistance is increasing.

Clostridium difficile (*C. diff*) is a Gram-positive anaerobic spore-forming bacteria. It is naturally present in the colon of around 5% of the adult population, and if normal gut flora is disrupted, for example, by antimicrobial therapy, it may result in *C. diff* infection. Enterotoxin-mediated colitis results in highly-infective diarrhoea, with high mortality in the elderly. The spores are not killed by alcohol gel and so nosocomial transmission is common. Moderate *C. diff* is treated with oral metronidazole, severe *C. diff* with oral vancomycin, and those at high risk of recurrence with fidaxomicin and consideration of IV immunoglobulin and a faecal transplant.

5) What is antimicrobial stewardship?

Antibiotic resistance is increasing, and is a worldwide problem. Antimicrobial stewardship is a program to promote the appropriate use of antimicrobial therapy in order to reduce resistance, decrease the spread of infection, and improve patient outcomes.
Features of antimicrobial stewardship programmes include:

- Restricted use of certain (usually broad-spectrum) antimicrobial agents, on the advice of a microbiology or intensive care specialist only. This prevents inappropriate use of last-line and broad-spectrum agents for infections that may be more appropriately treated using a narrow-spectrum agent.
- Daily review of antimicrobial prescriptions. Although early broad-spectrum therapy in severe infection is recommended in the treatment of sepsis and septic shock, these should be rationalised as soon as culture and sensitivity results are available, in order to use the appropriate agent with the narrowest spectrum of activity.
- Frequent (at least every week day) input from a microbiologist/infectious disease specialist, in order to review whether antimicrobial prescriptions are appropriate.
- Limitation of duration of antimicrobial therapy, according to clinical and biochemical markers of improvement, with appropriate conversion of intravenous agents to oral agents.
- Documentation of the indication of antimicrobial therapy and intended duration of action.

Summary of Key Points

- Sepsis and septic shock are frequently encountered in the critical care setting and carries a high mortality.
- The SOFA and qSOFA scores can be used to screen for organ dysfunction and possible sepsis.
- Early antimicrobial therapy, and then rationalisation using culture results with input from microbiologists, is best practice for preventing antimicrobial resistance.

References

1. Singer M, Deutschman CS, Seymour CW, *et al*. The third international consensus definitions for sepsis and septic shock (Sepsis-3). *JAMA* 2016; 315(8): 801-10.
2. Howell M, Davis A. Management of sepsis and septic shock. *JAMA* 2017; 317(8): 847-8.

Blunt thoracic trauma

1)   List the potential injuries for a patient with blunt thoracic trauma.

Blunt chest trauma is common and accounts for over 10% of admissions to the United Kingdom trauma network. There is of course the potential for injury to structures within the thoracic cage other than the lungs and chest wall — including damage to the heart and great vessels, oesophagus, spinal column and upper abdominal organs.

Chest injuries can be classified as occurring early or developing late as a complication of the initial trauma or the treatment provided, as outlined below.

Early injuries

- Traumatic pneumothorax or haemothorax which occurs at the time of injury and requires identification and drainage usually with a large-bore surgical chest drain.
- Tracheobronchial injury — rare, occurring in around 1% of cases, the severity depends on the level at which the injury occurs within the bronchial tree.
- Fractures, including:
  - sternal;
  - rib;
  - flail segments — where two or more adjacent ribs are fractured in two or more places causing paradoxical movement of that segment of the thoracic wall. This leads to ongoing pulmonary contusion and is extremely painful.
- Diaphragmatic damage or rupture — impairing ventilatory ability which may lead to respiratory failure.

Late complications

- Pulmonary contusions — typically develop after 24 hours and last for approximately 1 week.
- Hypoventilation — secondary to poor analgesia either as a result of fractures or interventions such as chest drains.
- Inability to clear secretions — usually secondary to pain with reduced tidal volumes and poor cough effort — may lead to lower respiratory tract infections.

2) Who is at risk of adverse outcomes from chest wall trauma?

Risk factors for adverse outcomes include:

- Increased number of rib fractures — although not a linear correlation there have been several studies which identified having five or more rib fractures visible on CT scanning leading to an adverse outcome independent of the other risk factors. If a single rib fracture was visible on chest X-ray (regardless of the number actually present on CT), then the same adverse outcome was observed.
- Increasing age — as with most conditions advanced age is associated with adverse outcomes even independent from comorbidity. It is likely that older patients who have less elasticity in their chest walls and more brittle bones will also suffer an increased number of rib fractures for the same applied force. Controlling for this, one study showed that in similar patients with four fractured ribs and an injury severity score of 11 who were intubated (for any reason), the mortality was 2.3% at age 50 but 19.8% at age 80.
- Comorbidity — a study in the United States showed that cardiovascular disease present prior to injury (coronary artery disease and heart failure) independently predicted poor outcome. Respiratory, renal or liver disease had no effect on the outcome observed in their population.

3)   What are the management priorities in chest wall trauma?

The goals when treating chest wall trauma can be classified:

- Analgesia — which can be provided systemically (opioid-based) or via regional anaesthesia (see below). There is no proven mortality benefit from regional anaesthesia over morphine but there is a trend towards improved analgesia and improved respiratory function. The aims of analgesia are to promote deep breathing and coughing, aiming to prevent the respiratory complications of chest wall injury.
- Respiratory support — there is no benefit to pre-emptively providing invasive or non-invasive respiratory support to this patient population. But the provision of humidified oxygen is recommended by the British Thoracic Society and the use of non-invasive support is as effective as invasive ventilation in the absence of any other indication to intubate the patient.
- Supportive measures — the mainstay of which is regular chest physiotherapy to aid secretion clearance. Some centres advocate the use of incentive spirometry as an exercise as well as to enable monitoring of respiratory function.

4)   What regional anaesthesia techniques are available for pain relief following chest wall injury?

There are four regional techniques described for chest wall analgesia, each of which have advantages and disadvantages:

- Thoracic epidural — the 'gold standard' technique in terms of efficacy of analgesia but it may be unhelpful in polytrauma where it may contribute to hypotension, mask intra-abdominal injury or be contraindicated by an acute coagulopathy of trauma.
- Thoracic paravertebral block — almost as efficacious as epidural anaesthesia and has the advantage of being able to target only the side affected if there are no bilateral injuries. There is less propensity

for cardiovascular instability and hypotension, and it is safer in a potentially coagulopathic patient but has an increased risk of pleural puncture and pneumothorax.

- Intercostal nerve blocks — less efficacious analgesia than the above methods and is commonly a single puncture rather than a continuous catheter technique. It involves multiple punctures if there are multiple rib fractures, so it can be potentially more distressing for the patient. It is relatively high risk in terms of local anaesthetic toxicity and inadvertent pleural puncture causing a pneumothorax.
- Intrapleural block — a less beneficial analgesic effect especially in the presence of an ipsilateral chest drain where as much as 50% of the local anaesthetic may be lost. There is a risk of introducing air and causing a pneumothorax. Patient position is important — they must be able to lie on their side (affected side uppermost) for a period of 10-15 minutes which may be difficult in the presence of bilateral injuries.

5) Who would benefit from operative rib fracture fixation following blunt thoracic trauma?

The two most recent trials on operative rib fixation both showed a reduced mortality, pneumonia rate and rate of tracheostomy insertion. These trials were conducted on patients with flail segments so it is difficult to extrapolate these results to non-flail segment chest injuries. A rib fracture consensus meeting recommended that those who should undergo operative fixation include:

- Those requiring a thoracotomy for any other reason.
- Those with pain uncontrolled by analgesia.
- Rib deformity greater than the diameter of the rib.
- Flail segments.
- Actual or impending respiratory failure or an inability to wean from ventilatory support.

The benefit of fixation is greatest if it occurs 48-72 hours after admission.

Summary of Key Points

- Chest wall trauma is common and causes considerable morbidity and mortality.
- Elderly patients with cardiovascular comorbidities who have multiple risk factors are most at risk of adverse outcomes.
- Analgesia is a key feature in the management of blunt chest trauma — both for patient comfort and to reduce complications.
- There are four recognised techniques of regional anaesthesia for rib fractures.
- Rib fixation should be considered early on a case-by-case basis.

References

1.   Livingston DH, Shogan B, John P, Lavery RF. CT Diagnosis of rib fractures and the prediction of acute respiratory failure. *J Trauma* 2008; 64(4): 905-11.

2.   Harrington DT, Phillips B, Machan J, *et al*; Research Consortium of New England Centers for Trauma (ReCONECT). Factors associated with survival following blunt chest trauma in older patients. *Arch Surg* 2010; 145(5): 432-7.

3.   Carrier FM, Turgeon AF, Nicole PC, *et al*. Effect of epidural analgesia in patients with traumatic rib fractures: a systematic review and meta-analysis of randomized controlled trials. *Can J Anesth* 2009; 56: 230-42.

4.   Gunduz M, Unlugenc H, Ozalevli M, *et al*. A comparative study of continuous positive airway pressure (CPAP) and intermittent positive pressure ventilation (IPPV) in patients with flail chest. *Emerg Med J* 2005; 22: 325-9.

5. Schuurmans J, Goslings JC, Schepers T. Operative management versus non-operative management of rib fractures in flail chest injuries: a systematic review. *Eur J Trauma Emerg Surg* 2017; 43(2): 163-8.

6. Slobogean GP, Kim H, Russell JP, *et al*. Rib fracture fixation restores inspiratory volume and peak flow in a full thorax human cadaveric breathing model. *Arch Trauma Res* 2015; 4(4): e28018.

Nutrition in intensive care

1)   Why is nutrition important in intensive care patients?

Although there is a lack of randomised controlled trials conclusively proving that intensive care unit nutrition is important, logic dictates that patients with critical illness have an ongoing need for calories to prevent catabolism and weakness with their potentially detrimental effect upon the duration of illness and outcome. The underlying nutritional science in critical illness remains poorly understood, but there are a few theories and goals described in the literature:

- The classic model of critical illness is characterised by catabolism exceeding anabolism and the recovery phase marked by the reversal of this — by providing nutritional support we provide substrate for anabolism and potentially trigger an earlier reversal of the catabolic processes.
- Fat mobilisation is poor during critical illness so carbohydrate substrate is especially important.
- Protein supplementation was thought to reduce the muscle breakdown observed during critical illness but the trials investigating this have been contradictory and indeed high levels of protein administration may worsen outcomes.

2)   What are the daily requirements of calories and the ratios of fat/protein/carbohydrate to make up this requirement?

The energy requirements of critically ill patients are notoriously difficult to assess and varies wildly depending upon the individual patient and the nature of their illness. There have been many attempts to use surrogate markers such as albumin and ferritin but these have proven to be unreliable in the context of illness.

The daily requirements of critically ill patients are as follows:

- Calorific requirement is thought to be in the region of 25-30kcal/kg/day, steadily increased from an initial starting rate of 8-10kcal/kg/day.
- Protein requirements vary depending upon the severity of critical illness, based upon studies of nitrogen balance. Current recommendations are 1-1.5g/kg/day for most patients, increasing to 1.5-2g/kg/day in patients with severe catabolic illnesses such as burns.
- Carbohydrate is the next most important as it is the body's preferred energy substrate in critical illness. It should make up at least 50% of the remaining calorie requirement after protein, usually at a level of 3-4g/kg/day.
- Fat/lipids make up the rest of the requirement and, while its role as an energy substrate in critical illness is unclear, it certainly has a role in cellular homeostasis and immune function.
- Other considerations include the need for electrolytes and micronutrients, some of the daily requirements of which are:
  - sodium — 1-2mmol/kg/day;
  - potassium — 0.7-1mmol/kg/day;
  - calcium — 0. 1mmol/kg/day;
  - magnesium — 0.1mmol/kg/day;
  - phosphate — 0.4mmol/kg/day;
  - vitamin C — 90mg/day;
  - folic acid — 400μg/day.

Expert input from a critical care dietitian is recommended to aid decision-making surrounding the provision of nutritional support.

3) When might parenteral nutrition be appropriate?

Generally, enteral nutrition is the first-line option in most intensive care units due to its lower cost and infection rate, and the lack of the need for ongoing central venous access. However, there are certain circumstances where enteral nutrition is not appropriate:

- Gastrointestinal tract failure — may be secondary to ileus post-laparotomy, inflammatory disease flare-ups, hypoperfusion, drugs or infections within the GI tract itself.
- Loss of gastrointestinal tract length and therefore an inability to absorb sufficient nutrition to support the calorific requirements.

There have been several trials comparing early versus late use of parenteral nutrition with conflicting results. One showed that early parenteral nutrition reduced the duration of mechanical ventilation whilst another showed that early initiation of parenteral nutrition increased ICU and hospital stay whilst delaying for 7 days had no detrimental effect on mortality.

Pragmatically, it is recommended to consider the nutritional needs of patients on an individual basis and consider parenteral nutrition when the enteral route is unlikely to be effective within the first 7-10 days of their illness.

4) What complications are associated with parenteral nutrition?

The complications related to parenteral nutrition can be classified as below.

- Associated with central venous access including:
    - insertion complications — damage to other structures, pneumothorax;
    - the need for ongoing and long duration of lines — increased risk of catheter-associated thrombosis and catheter-associated infections/colonisation.

- Infective:
  - patients with a central line receiving parenteral nutrition are at a higher risk of bacterial and fungal blood stream infections compared to those with a central line who are not receiving parenteral nutrition. This is likely as a result of the nutrition solution being an ideal growth medium for pathogenic organisms.
- Metabolic:
  - glucose — hyperglycaemia is common with parenteral nutrition and an insulin infusion is often required alongside. Conversely, rebound hypoglycaemia occurs on cessation of parenteral nutrition even without exogenous insulin infusions;
  - micronutrient deficiencies — these need to be routinely monitored and replaced if patients are on parenteral nutrition for a prolonged period of time;
  - lipaemia — which may interfere with routine blood tests and can cause acute pancreatitis;
  - liver abnormalities including cholestasis which is dose- and duration of parental nutrition-dependent and usually benign.

5) Is there a role for L-arginine as an immune-enhancing nutritional agent in intensive care?

Normally a non-essential amino acid, L-arginine becomes essential during times of metabolic stress such as critical illness. It is thought to upregulate the inflammatory response and the action of phagocytes. There is some evidence that supplementation with L-arginine therefore reduces infective complications and promotes wound healing after elective surgery but it is insufficient to recommend its routine use as a supplement in the critically ill population.

Summary of Key Points

- Nutritional support is important in the critically unwell population, especially those with highly catabolic conditions such as burns.
- Calorific and other nutrient requirements have generic recommended regimes but should be considered on a case-by-case basis with the help of an expert dietitian.
- Protein supplementation is crucial, especially in highly catabolic states.
- Parenteral nutrition may be required but is more expensive and associated with more complications than enteral nutrition.
- There is no clearly defined role for routine L-arginine supplementation in the intensive care unit.

References

1.   Marik PE, Zaloga GP. Early enteral nutrition in acutely ill patients: a systematic review. *Crit Care Med* 2001; 29: 2264.

2.   Dvir D, Cohen J, Singer P. Computerized energy balance and complications in critically ill patients: an observational study. *Clin Nutr* 2006; 25: 37.

3.   Casaer MP, Wilmer A, Hermans G, *et al*. Role of disease and macronutrient dose in the randomized controlled EPaNIC trial: a post hoc analysis. *Am J Respir Crit Care Med* 2013; 187: 247.

4.   Doig GS, Simpson F, Sweetman EA, *et al*. Early parenteral nutrition in critically ill patients with short-term relative contraindications to early enteral nutrition: a randomized controlled trial. *JAMA* 2013; 309(20): 2130-8.

5.   Casaer MP, Mesotten D, Hermans G, *et al*. Early vs. late parenteral nutrition. *N Engl J Med* 2011; 365(6): 506-17.

6.   Kritchevsky SB, Braun BI, Kusek L, *et al*. The impact of hospital practice on central venous catheter associated bloodstream infection rates at the patient and unit level: a multicenter study. *Am J Med Qual* 2008; 23: 24.

7.   Kalil AC, Danner RL. L-Arginine supplementation in sepsis: beneficial or harmful? *Curr Opin Crit Care* 2006; 12: 303.

SET 6

Circulatory assist devices

1) A) What is the purpose of ventricular assist devices (VADs)?

- VADs are mechanical systems which support the left ventricle (LVAD), right ventricle (RVAD), or both (BIVAD), reducing myocardial work whilst maintaining cardiac output and vital organ perfusion.

B) What are the indications for a VAD?

- A bridge to recovery or heart transplantation in acute heart failure/cardiogenic shock, e.g.:
  - myocardial infarction;
  - myocardial stunning post-cardiac surgery;
  - viral cardiomyopathy.
- A bridge therapy whilst awaiting (or destination therapy in those inappropriate for) heart transplantation in advanced chronic heart failure refractory to medical therapy, e.g.:
  - coronary artery disease;
  - hypertensive heart disease;
  - ischaemic and dilated cardiomyopathies.
- The aim for long-term therapy is for LVAD support alone; RV failure often improves with LVAD implantation. True biventricular failure requiring BIVAD has a worse prognosis.

C) List some contraindications to VAD implantation.

Cardiovascular

- Biventricular failure >65 years old.
- Severe mitral or aortic valve disease unamenable to correction.
- Abdominal aortic aneurysm >5cm.

Respiratory

- Severe respiratory disease (FEV$_1$ <1L).
- Fixed pulmonary hypertension.

Renal

- Long-term dialysis.
- Serum creatinine >265µmol/L.

Hepatic

- Cirrhosis.
- Fixed portal hypertension.

Neuropsychological

- Recent/evolving stroke.
- Severe neurological deficit.
- Significant psychiatric disease.
- Inadequate psychosocial support.

Haematological

- Contraindication to anticoagulation.
- Heparin-induced thrombocytopenia.

Microbiological

- Severe sepsis.
- Immunodeficiency.

Malignancy

- Metastatic cancer.

Nutritional

- Morbid obesity (BMI >40).
- Chronic severe malnutrition (BMI <20).

2) Outline the various technologies used for circulatory assistance.

- VADs are inserted via a median sternotomy or left thoracotomy with the LVAD inserted from the left atrium or ventricle to the ascending aorta, the RVAD from the right atrium or ventricle to the main pulmonary artery.
- Short-term devices have an extracorporeal pump.
- Long-term devices have an implanted pump, with a driveline, battery packs and operating console externally, and may allow patient discharge home.
- Pumps can be pulsatile- or continuous-flow, with axial-flow or centrifugal pumping, with or without bearings.
- VADs require anticoagulation, although bearingless systems require less intense anticoagulation.
- Intra-aortic balloon pump (IABP) counterpulsation, the Impella® circulatory support system, and peripheral veno-arterial extracorporeal membrane oxygenation (ECMO) are alternative short-term therapies.
- An IABP can be utilised in addition to an LVAD to augment left ventricular function.

- ECMO, although requiring intensive resources, provides both heart and lung support without the need for a sternotomy.
- Technology also exists for explanation of the native heart and replacement with a total artificial heart.

3) What is an intra-aortic balloon pump (IABP)?

- IABP counterpulsation is a short-term coronary and systemic perfusion assist device.
- It is indicated to help achieve haemodynamic stability in:
  - acute myocardial infarction;
  - cardiogenic shock;
  - unstable angina;
  - refractory ventricular failure;
  - post-cardiac surgery.
- It is a catheter with an integral balloon of various sizes inserted percutaneously usually via the femoral artery into the descending aorta, with the tip lying 1-2cm distal to the origin of the left subclavian artery.
- The catheter is connected to a console with ECG or an arterial pressure waveform used to time the pump counterpulsation to inflate the balloon with helium during diastole and deflate in systole. Helium is used to reduce the risk associated with gas embolism if the balloon ruptures but also for its low density to promote laminar flow and faster inflation and deflation of the balloon.
- It aims to improve ventricular performance by augmenting coronary perfusion and therefore myocardial oxygen supply during diastole, with balloon deflation in systole reducing myocardial oxygen demand by reducing left ventricular afterload.
- IABP is prothrombotic so patients should be anticoagulated.
- It is possible for the catheter to migrate and compromise subclavian, common carotid or renal arteries, in addition to other complications such as vascular trauma and haematological abnormalities, so vigilance is required.

4) What is an Impella®?

- An Impella® is an alternative short-term, minimally invasive, catheter-based assist device indicated for acute heart failure/cardiogenic shock.
- It is inserted via the femoral artery with the tip crossing the aortic valve to rest in the left ventricle.
- It has an inlet area near the tip, with blood pumped from the left ventricle across the aortic valve and via the outlet into the ascending aorta.
- It acts to unload the left ventricle, maintaining organ perfusion and allows recovery of the native heart.

5) List some common problems encountered in the postoperative ICU care of VAD implantation patients.

Bleeding

- Coagulopathy and postoperative bleeding are common. Early re-exploration should be considered. Transfusion should be guided by thromboelastography and laboratory results.

Cardiac tamponade

- Signs include:
  - reduced VAD flows;
  - rising CVP;
  - reduced MAP;
  - escalating inotropic requirements;
  - metabolic acidosis;
  - oliguria.
- Requires immediate surgical decompression.

Haemodynamic instability

- Causes include:
  - right ventricular dysfunction;
  - underfilling;
  - cardiac tamponade (see above).
- Continuous postoperative use of transoesophageal echocardiography aids in determining the cause and aiding management.

Fluid overload

- Secondary to significant blood product transfusion or mobilisation of oedema.
- Haemofiltration is indicated if cardiovascularly stable.

Vasoplegia

- Secondary to phosphodiesterase inhibitors or systemic inflammatory response syndrome (SIRS).
- Norepinephrine and vasopressin may be indicated to maintain organ perfusion.

Gastrointestinal and hepatic dysfunction

- Ileus is a common postoperative finding, managed with prokinetics.
- Liver dysfunction is common in patients with chronic heart failure.

Infection

- Antibiotic prophylaxis according to local policy.
- With VADs being a foreign body and patients often with a pre-operative susceptibility to infection, high vigilance and appropriate management of postoperative infection are required.

Summary of Key Points

- Circulatory assist devices include short- or long-term (left, right, and bi-) ventricular assist devices, intra-aortic balloon pump counterpulsation, the Impella® circulatory support system, ECMO and artificial hearts.
- In principle, the technologies aim to assist appropriately selected patients with acute or chronic heart failure and cardiogenic shock by supplementing the myocardial pump with artificial pumping, thereby reducing myocardial work, maintaining cardiac output and vital organ perfusion.
- Circulatory assist devices are not without complications and vigilance is required by the appropriately trained critical care teams caring for these complex patients.

References

1. Harris P, Kuppurao L. Ventricular assist devices. *Contin Educ Anaesth Crit Care Pain* 2012; 12(3): 145-51.
2. Krishna M, Zacharowski K. Principles of intra-aortic balloon pump counterpulsation. *Contin Educ Anaesth Crit Care Pain* 2009; 9(1): 24-8.

Pancreatitis

1) What is pancreatitis and what are its causes?

Pancreatitis refers to inflammation of the pancreas. It may be acute or chronic. Causes of acute pancreatitis are listed below, and can be remembered using the mnemonic "GET SMASHED":

- **G**allstones.
- **E**thanol.
- **T**rauma/burns/surgery.
- **S**teroids.
- **M**umps/infective.
- **A**utoimmune.
- **S**corpion bite.
- **H**yperlipidaemia/hypercalcaemia/hyperparathyroidism.
- **E**ndoscopic retrograde cholangiopancreatography (ERCP).
- **D**rugs — for example, pentamidine, azathioprine.
- Malignancy.
- Pregnancy.

Gallstones, ethanol and trauma are the most common causes. Smoking has recently been implicated as an independent risk factor for the development of pancreatitis.

2) Can you classify acute pancreatitis?

The revised Atlanta classification (2012) divides pancreatitis into mild, moderate and severe (● Table 6.1). Critical pancreatitis is a more recent concept applied to infected pancreatic necrosis with persistent organ failure.

Table 6.1. Revised Atlanta Classification.

Mild	No organ failure, no local or systemic complications
Moderate	Transient organ failure (<48 hours) or local or systemic complications
Severe	Persistent organ failure >48 hours' duration

Local complications include pancreatic pseudocyst formation, peripancreatic fluid accumulation and necrosis.

Severe pancreatitis has a mortality of around 30%.

Systemic inflammatory response syndrome (SIRS) frequently develops in severe pancreatitis, resulting in shock, pulmonary oedema and acute respiratory distress syndrome (ARDS).

The modified Glasgow Score (● Table 6.2) can be used to identify those that may benefit from critical care admission.

Table 6.2. Modified Glasgow Score.

PaO_2	<7.9kPa
Age	>55 years
WBC	>15 x 10^9/L
Calcium	<2mmol/L
Urea	>16mmol/L
LDH	>600 IU/L
Albumin	<32g/L
Blood glucose	>10mmol/L

Each point scores 1. A score of 3 or more is associated with a mortality of 15% and should be referred to critical care.

3) What is the role of diagnostic imaging in patients with pancreatitis?

Radiological criteria exist to classify pancreatitis. Diagnostic criteria for pancreatitis include two of the following: abdominal pain, raised serum amylase or lipase greater than three times the upper limit of normal, or characteristic findings on imaging.

Contrast-enhanced CT is of use in establishing disease severity, although clinical indicators are equally validated in early disease. Early CT is therefore only useful when there is diagnostic uncertainty. Sequential CT, every 7 to 10 days, is useful in establishing progression or resolution of inflammation, pseudocyst and necrosis.

4) Outline the critical care management of patients with severe pancreatitis.

General supportive measures should be established. Supplemental oxygen therapy has a proven mortality benefit in patients with severe pancreatitis.

Pain control can be problematic and a multimodal approach to analgesia is recommended.

Hypotension and hypovolaemia are common and a balanced crystalloid solution should be used to establish intravascular volume. In fluid-refractory hypotension, noradrenaline should be started as a first-line vasopressor. Cardiac output monitoring may be of benefit.

Respiratory failure may develop either as a consequence of diaphragmatic splinting and pain, or acute respiratory distress syndrome. High-flow nasal oxygenation, non-invasive ventilation or invasive ventilation should be established as appropriate.

Early nutritional support should be established. Post-pyloric feeding with a nasojejunal tube may be preferred over nasogastric feeding. Parenteral nutrition may be required if absorption from the gastrointestinal tract is poor. Hyperglycaemia is common and should be treated with an intravenous insulin infusion.

In pancreatic necrosis, antimicrobial therapy alone may be sufficient, but if not, necrosectomy via open, laparoscopic or endoscopic (transgastric) techniques may be used.

Summary of Key Points

- Pancreatitis is a common presentation to general intensive care, often requiring advanced organ support.
- A modified Glasgow Score >3 warrants critical care review.
- Supplemental oxygen and early feeding have a proven mortality benefit in patients with pancreatitis.
- Antibiotics alone can be effective in treating pancreatic necrosis.

References

1.   Lankisch PG, Apte M, Banks PA. Acute pancreatitis. *Lancet* 2015; 386: 85-96.

Drowning

1) Can you classify drowning into subtypes?

Drowning is defined as submersion/immersion in water and is subclassified into four subtypes (● Table 6.3).

Table 6.3. Classification of drowning.	
Class 1	No evidence of inhalation of water
Class 2	Evidence of inhalation of water and adequate ventilation
Class 3	Evidence of inhalation of water and inadequate ventilation
Class 4	Absent ventilation and circulation

2) What are the risk factors associated with drowning?

Risk factors can be considered as those inherent to the patient and those associated with the activity surrounding the drowning incident.

Patient risk factors

- Seizure disorders — and the onset of a seizure whilst in or around water.
- Undetected primary cardiac arrhythmias — for example, Type 1 long QT syndrome which can trigger arrhythmias, especially in conjunction with cold water immersion and strenuous exercise.

- Inability to swim, or overestimation of swimming ability.
- Underlying ischaemic heart disease.

Activity-related risk factors

- Underestimation of the water conditions/tide/current/temperature.
- Use of alcohol or illicit drugs.
- Risk-taking/showing-off behaviour.
- Inadequate supervision of children.
- Trauma upon entering the water, for example, shallow diving hitting the floor or an underwater obstacle not appreciated before entry.
- Rapid shallow breathing before entry to the water — used as a technique to prolong dive duration. This leads to a low partial pressure of carbon dioxide in the blood. Whilst underwater, oxygen is consumed but the carbon dioxide does not rise quickly enough to trigger the urge to breathe, therefore the subject is hypoxaemic but not hypercapnic. This may lead to seizures and loss of consciousness.

3) What pathophysiological effects occur as a result of water inhalation?

Water inhalation usually follows a period of general panic, struggling to remain above the water and an abnormal breathing pattern. A reflex inspiratory effort is eventually triggered, which then causes hypoxia via the following mechanisms:

- Laryngospasm when water hits the laryngeal inlet or as a reflex once it enters the lower respiratory tract.
- Aspiration of water into the lower respiratory tract reducing the surface area of the lungs available for gaseous exchange, leading to ventilation/perfusion mismatching as well as directly causing a reduction in lung compliance.

- Surfactant is washed out by both fresh and salt water — this leads to non-cardiogenic pulmonary oedema and may be a trigger for ARDS.

Other organ system effects include:

- Cardiovascular — arrhythmias (usually secondary to hypoxaemia and hypothermia).
- Neurological — within 24 hours there may be an acute rise in intracranial pressure secondary to hypoxic ischaemic damage causing cerebral oedema.
- Metabolic — usually a mixed respiratory and metabolic acidosis. This is less likely to cause acute disturbances of electrolytes unless associated with renal failure or drowning in special media, e.g. the Dead Sea.

4) How should patients be managed following drowning?

Pre-hospital management

- The casualty should be removed from the water and assessed with an 'airway, breathing, circulation, disability and exposure' approach. If possible, the rescuer should not enter the water and only do so as a last resort — if they do enter the water, a floatation aid must be taken.
- The risk of spinal injury with drowning is low unless there is concomitant trauma or the victim is known to have dived head first into shallow water.
- Where possible, victims should be removed from the water horizontally to prevent cardiovascular collapse.
- If required, advanced life support (ALS) should be initiated — early initiation post-drowning has been shown to improve outcome. Note, the drowning ALS algorithm differs from the standard adult cardiac

arrest algorithm as it prioritises ventilation over chest compressions — including the use of five rescue breaths initially (supplemented with oxygen if available).

- If defibrillation is required, ensure that the patient's chest is dry before applying the pads and make sure rescuers are not in contact with the patient via a pool of water before defibrillation.
- Attempt to prevent further cooling with the use of blankets and removal of wet clothes.

Emergency department management

- Continue the pre-hospital resuscitation.
- Supplemental oxygen, secure the airway with an endotracheal tube (ETT) if required.
- If intubated, insert a gastric tube to empty the stomach — water ingestion is common and may impair ventilation even in adult drowning victims.
- If the drowning occurred in cold water, then a prolonged resuscitation may be indicated along with rewarming to 32-35°C. Consider the use of a mechanical chest compression device and a low-reading thermometer. Neurological outcome is likely to be poor if return of spontaneous circulation does not occur within 30 minutes of advanced life support, although case reports exist of remarkable survival after prolonged submersion and protracted resuscitation, especially in children and cold water.
- In less severe cases, supplemental oxygen and admission for monitoring are indicated. All patients who develop symptoms after immersion do so within 7 hours, so a period of observation may be indicated.

Intensive care management

- Neurological issues — predominantly cerebral oedema leading to raised intracranial pressure. Treat as per a head injury and use secondary brain injury prevention methods (blood pressure management, osmotherapy, ventilator care bundles, ensure adequate oxygenation and normocarbia, maintenance of euglycaemia and control of seizures).

- The use of therapeutic hypothermia remains controversial and the avoidance of hyperthermia, as with a standard out-of-hospital cardiac arrest, is recommended.
- Ventilation should be as per the standard "ARDSnet" protocols. There is no role for prophylactic antibiotics, but they should be commenced if there is evidence of infection. There is no evidence to support the use of steroids or exogenous surfactant in drowning patients in the ICU.
- Cardiovascular instability can be due to significant hypovolaemia (during submersion, vasoconstriction shunts blood to the core and reduces antidiuretic hormone production) or hypoxic myocardial damage/stunning. Careful assessment of the cardiovascular system is required at regular intervals during rewarming. Patients may require significant amounts of fluid as well as inotropic or vasopressor support.

5) What information can be used to aid prognostication following submersion injury?

The submersion time is the most critical factor when attempting to prognosticate after a submersion injury and indeed it plays a role in rescue operations as well, with the rescue services reviewing operations at 30 and 60 minutes after their arrival, with operations usually ceasing at the 90-minute point and changing to recovery operations. These decisions are based upon the patient and the water temperature as well as the risk to the rescuers. Prolonged operations are more likely in good conditions with cold water and a paediatric victim.

The following factors are linked to poor prognosis if present at presentation:

- Age >14.
- Submersion >5 minutes.
- Time to basic life support >10 minutes.
- 25 minutes of resuscitation without return of spontaneous circulation.
- GCS <5.
- Arterial pH <7.1.

Summary of Key Points

- There are four drowning subtypes.
- Many drowning victims are under the influence of drugs and/or alcohol and this is the major modifiable risk factor.
- The ingestion of water has significant impact upon all the organ systems.
- Patients should be managed as per the Resuscitation Council guidelines for pre-hospital arrests, with greater emphasis on oxygenation and ventilation when compared with standard adult resuscitation algorithms.
- The duration of submersion has the greatest impact upon rescue attempts and subsequent prognosis.

References

1.   Salomez F, Vincent JL. Drowning: a review of epidemiology, pathophysiology, treatment and prevention. *Resuscitation* 2004; 63: 261.

2.   Bierens JJ, Knape JT, Gelissen HP. Drowning. *Curr Opin Crit Care* 2002; 8: 578.

3.   Yagil Y, Stalnikowicz R, Michaeli J, Mogle P. Near drowning in the dead sea. Electrolyte imbalances and therapeutic implications. *Arch Intern Med* 1985; 145: 50.

4.   Resuscitation Council (UK) adult resuscitation guidelines - prehospital resuscitation. Available from: www.resus.org.uk.

5.   Venema AM, Groothoff JW, Bierens JJ. The role of bystanders during rescue and resuscitation of drowning victims. *Resuscitation* 2010; 81: 434.

6.   Causey AL, Tilelli JA, Swanson ME. Predicting discharge in uncomplicated near-drowning. *Am J Emerg Med* 2000; 18: 9.

7.   Choi SP, Youn CS, Park KN, *et al*. Therapeutic hypothermia in adult cardiac arrest because of drowning. *Acta Anaesthesiol Scand* 2012; 56: 116.

8.   Quan L, Bierens JJ, Lis R, *et al*. Predicting outcome of drowning at the scene: a systematic review and meta-analyses. *Resuscitation* 2016; 104: 63.

Organ donation

1) What categories of solid organ donation are you aware of?

There are three types of solid organ donation:

- Donation after a patient has met the criteria for brain stem death (donation after brainstem death [DBD]).
- Donation after circulatory death (DCD) when a patient's heart has stopped and it is inappropriate to resuscitate them. This also applies to donation after a patient has died subsequent to withdrawal of life-sustaining treatment in the intensive care unit. This type of organ donation can be further subclassified:
  - category 1 — dead on arrival — uncontrolled;
  - category 2 — unsuccessful resuscitation — uncontrolled;
  - category 3 — anticipated cardiac arrest — controlled, usually after withdrawal of life-sustaining treatment;
  - category 4 — cardiac arrest in a brain-dead patient awaiting donation — controlled;
  - category 5 — unexpected cardiac arrest on intensive care — uncontrolled.

  Clearly the most commonly used DCD is category 3. Categories 1, 2 and 5 are usually only an option if they occur in a transplant centre.
- Living donation — most commonly when a living person donates one of their kidneys or a small part of their liver to be used by another person.

2)   What contraindications may prevent organ donation?

There are some general contraindications and then some organ-specific contraindications to be considered before the process of referral for organ donation.

General contraindications

- Age >85.
- Primary intracerebral lymphoma.
- All secondary intracerebral tumours.
- Any active cancer with spread outside the primary organ within the last 3 years, i.e. not in remission and includes local spread to lymph nodes.
- Active haematological malignancy.
- Definite, probable or possible transmissible spongiform encephalopathy.
- Active or untreated tuberculosis.
- HIV disease manifestation (HIV infected patients may still donate their organs to appropriately counselled HIV infected recipients).
- History of Ebola virus infection.

Organ-specific contraindications

Organ-specific contraindications pertain to the individual organ only, so other organs can be used from patients who have specific organs excluded by the below contraindications:

- Liver — cirrhosis, acute viral hepatitis, ALT >10,000 IU/L, portal venous thrombosis.
- Bowel — cannot be used from DCD donors at all or DBD donors who are aged 56 or older or who weigh 80kg or more, or who have underlying chronic intestinal disease, e.g. Crohn's disease.

- Kidney — chronic kidney disease stage 3B or worse, eGFR <45ml/min/1.73m^2, chronic renal dialysis patient.
- Pancreas — diabetes mellitus of any type, BMI >40, DBD donors aged 66 or older, DCD donors aged 56 or older.
- Heart — documented coronary artery disease, LV ejection fraction <30% on more than one occasion of imaging, massive inotropic or vasopressor support with adequate intravascular filling.
- Lungs — chest X-ray evidence of massive consolidation, significant chronic lung disease (excluding controlled asthma), DCD donors aged 65 or older, DBD donors aged 70 or older.

3) What are the criteria for diagnosing brainstem death?

There are criteria set down in a code of practice published by the Academy of Medical Royal Colleges which govern the diagnosis of brainstem death. There are a group of preconditions, a set of rules concerning the tests and then the tests themselves.

Preconditions

- There must be irreversible brain damage of known aetiology — this can be a primary intracranial cause, e.g. haemorrhage, or as a result of an extracranial event, e.g. prolonged hypoxaemia which has then caused damage to the brain and brainstem.
- The cause of coma and apnoea must not be as a result of the following:
  - neuromuscular blockade — this is excluded by the presence of deep tendon reflexes as well as testing with nerve stimulation devices;
  - deep sedation — consideration of the sedative drugs used, their doses and duration of administration, along with the patient's renal and hepatic function should be undertaken and

sufficient time allowed for the effect of these drugs to wear off. Drug levels may be appropriate, especially for thiopentone which may persist for a long time (a level of <5mg/L is required to enable testing to go ahead). If the cause of coma may be as a result of a sedative medication for which there is an antidote, then this should be administered to confirm that it is not contributing to the low conscious level and loss of cerebral function, e.g. naloxone for opioids;

- hypothermia — brainstem function may be lost in patients whose core body temperature is <28°C. Mildly hypothermic patients (32-34°C) may also have impaired consciousness. Brainstem tests cannot therefore be undertaken unless the patient has a core temperature consistent with being conscious, i.e. >34°C;

- the patient's mean arterial pressure must be above 60mmHg, with a $PaCO_2$ <6kPa, PaO_2 >10kPa and a pH between 7.35-7.45 to ensure that there is no cardiorespiratory cause of the loss of consciousness;

- the metabolic function of the patient should be as near normal as possible — this includes a normal blood glucose >3mmol/L but <20mmol/L. It is uncommon for conditions such as profound hypothyroidism or an Addisonian crisis to exist alongside the known severe brain injury, so they may be considered if there is objective evidence of their presence, but routine monitoring of hormone assays is not required;

- the serum sodium must be >115mmol/L and less than 160mmol/L with the understanding that the trend, rate of development or rate of correction of a serum sodium must be taken into account by looking at the recent blood tests. Similarly, abnormalities of serum potassium, magnesium or phosphate levels may be associated with profound weakness and should be maintained in the following ranges prior to testing:

- ■ potassium >2mmol/L;
- ■ magnesium >0.5mmol/L but <3mmol/L;
- ■ phosphate >0.5mmol/L but <3mmol/L.
- High cervical spine injury must be excluded in patients with head injury to ensure that this is not the cause of their apnoea.

Testing

This must be carried out by two suitably trained doctors both of whom have been fully registered with the General Medical Council for more than 5 years, one of whom must be a consultant. They must not have (or be perceived to have) any conflict of interest concerning the case and neither may be part of the transplant team. Two sets of tests are conducted but there is no set time period that needs to be observed between tests. The legal time of death is the time at which the first set of tests are complete, if they have shown complete loss of brainstem function. The second set of tests is then used to confirm this diagnosis with absolute certainty.

The following tests of brainstem function are then undertaken:

- The pupils must be fixed in diameter and not change in size with a light stimulus (cranial nerves II and III).
- There must be no corneal reflex when stimulated with a soft cloth/cotton wool (cranial nerves V and VII).
- There is no vestibulo-ocular reflex — with clear external auditory canals, at least 50ml ice cold water is slowly injected to come into contact with each ear drum over a period of 1 minute (cranial nerves VIII and III).
- There is no motor response to a painful stimulus of the supraorbital ridge — either in the cranial nerve distribution or with limb movement (cranial nerves V and VII).
- There is no gag reflex in response to stimulation of the posterior pharyngeal wall with a spatula or Yankauer suction tube (cranial nerve IX).

- There is no cough reflex to bronchial stimulation achieved by passing a suction catheter down the endotracheal tube (cranial nerve X).
- The last test is the apnoea test (to prevent harm by hypoxia if other tests do not confirm brainstem death prior to reaching this stage). N.B. the previous testing must occur with a normal $PaCO_2$ level (<6kPa) which should only be allowed to rise to >6kPa (with a pH <7.4) once they have been completed. The patient is then disconnected from the ventilator with oxygenation continuing via a catheter placed within the endotracheal tube and connected to an oxygen supply. The patient is observed for respiratory effort for a period of 5 minutes — if there is none then a rise in $PaCO_2$ of more than 0.5kPa is confirmed with an ABG. The patient must then be ventilated back to a normal $PaCO_2$ prior to the commencement of the second set of tests.

4) What physiological changes occur after brainstem death?

The loss of brainstem autoregulation has a profound effect on all body systems and if a patient is left without intervention then brainstem death would inevitably be followed by cardiac death.

These effects include:

- Cardiovascular — hypotension as a result of the loss of sympathetic tone combined with the potential hypovolaemia secondary to cranial diabetes insipidus — both should be treated with volume replacement and cardiovascular support in terms of inotropes and vasopressors to support organ perfusion if transplantation is being considered.
- Metabolic — diabetes insipidus commonly develops and should be treated with desmopressin. Other abnormalities may include profound functional hypothyroidism and hypothermia.

199

- Coagulation — coagulopathies may result from platelet dysfunction secondary to catecholamine release as well as tissue plasminogen activating factor and thromboplastin as a direct consequence of damage to brain tissue.

5) What are the time limitations applied to donation after cardiac death?

To limit the functional warm ischaemic time of organs to be harvested for DCD, it often appears more rushed than the DBD donation process. In particular, it is important throughout the discussion with the patient's family that they understand that once their loved one dies they will only remain on the intensive care unit for approximately 5 minutes after they have died — during which time the doctor who is going to confirm cardiac death will observe the patient and confirm death in the normal manner. The patient will then be rapidly transferred to the operating theatre to ensure that the organs to be harvested remain viable.

In addition, there are limits to the functional warm ischaemic time that are organ-specific:

- Kidney — 120 minutes — although this can be extended by up to another 120 minutes if it is thought that the organ may still be viable in specific circumstances.
- Liver — 30 minutes — DCD livers have a higher incidence of graft failure than DBD hence the short tolerance of functional warm ischaemic time.
- Lung — 60 minutes — although the time to reinflation of the lungs is more important than the functional warm ischaemic time.
- Pancreas — 30 minutes.

Summary of Key Points

- There are various types of solid organ donation: DBD, DCD and living donation.
- Exclusion criteria are complex — if in doubt, consult with your local specialist nurse for organ donation.
- Diagnosis of brainstem death has rigid criteria.
- Complex physiology occurs after brainstem death.
- DCD has more stringent time pressures than DBD in terms of minimising the warm ischaemic time of the organs to be harvested.

References

1. Zalewska K. Clinical contraindications for approaching families for possible organ donation. NHS organ donation and transplant policy 188/5.2. Available from: http://www.odt.nhs.uk/pdf/contraindications_to_organ_donation.pdf.

2. Academy of Medical Royal Colleges. A code of practice for the diagnosis and confirmation of death, 2008. Available from: http://aomrc.org.uk/wp-content/uploads/2016/04/Code_Practice_Confirmation_Diagnosis_Death_1008-4.pdf.

3. Gordon JK, McKinlay J. Physiological changes after brain stem death and management of the heart-beating donor. *Contin Educ Anaesth Crit Care Pain* 2012; 12(5): 225-9.

4. Department of Health. Organ donation after circulatory death. Report of a consensus meeting. Intensive Care Society, NHS Blood and Transplant, and British Transplantation Society, 2010. Available from: http://www.ics.ac.uk/intensive_care_professional/standards_ and_guidelines/dcd.

Mental capacity and deprivation of liberty in intensive care

1) Briefly outline the underlying key principles of the Mental Capacity Act (2005) England and Wales.

There are five key principles on which the Mental Capacity Act (MCA) is based:

- Every adult has the right to make his or her own decisions and must be assumed to have capacity to do so unless it is proved otherwise.
- People must be supported as much as possible to make and communicate their decision before anyone concludes that they are unable to do so; for example, a letter board may be used to aid patients who are unable to communicate verbally (e.g. tracheostomy ventilated) in letting their wishes be known. This consists of a board containing groups of letters to enable the patient to spell out words with either their finger or using eye movements. It can be a slow process and frustrating for everyone involved but is nevertheless important.
- People have the right to make what others might regard as unwise or eccentric decisions.
- Anything done for or on behalf of a person who lacks mental capacity must be done in their best interests.
- Before the act is done, or the decision made, regard must be had to whether the purpose for which it is needed can be as effectively achieved in a way that is less restrictive of the person's rights and freedom of action.

2) When assessing a patient's capacity to make a decision, what four prerequisites are they required to demonstrate?

- Understand information about the decision to be made.
- Retain that information in their mind.

- Use or weigh that information as part of the decision-making process.
- Communicate their decision.

3) A) What principle is used to determine the approach to treatment and decisions made on behalf of a patient who lacks capacity?

- Where a patient lacks capacity for a particular medical treatment decision (and there is no effective advance decision to refuse treatment [ADRT] to predetermine this), then a best interests decision must be made.
- The lead clinician responsible for the patient is likely to be the decision maker and should take a collaborative approach to determining the patient's best interests, including social and emotional aspects in addition to medical ones, informed by the patient's own wishes, feelings, beliefs and values.

B) Who can give consent or refuse treatment on behalf of an incapacitated patient?

- Those with a lasting power of attorney (England and Wales) or welfare attorney (Scotland) appointed by the patient.
- Court of Protection appointed deputies.

C) Who should be consulted when considering a patient's best interests?

In addition to attorneys and deputies:

- Anyone named by the patient as someone they want to be consulted.
- Anyone involved in caring for the person.

- Anyone interested in their welfare, e.g. family, friends.
- An independent mental capacity advocate (IMCA), if there is no one else to speak to about the patient's best interests.

D) What approach would you take when resolving a dispute between your proposed course of action for a patient and the opinion of those close to the patient?

- If possible, delay any proposed course of action, e.g. allow delirium to resolve and the patient to regain capacity.
- Involve the Patient Advocacy and Liaison Service (PALS).
- Seek a second opinion from an impartial clinician.
- Involve an independent advocate such as an IMCA.
- Hold a case conference.
- Involve mediation services.
- Seek legal advice; ultimately the Court of Protection may need to make a final decision.

E) What approach should be taken with the care of a patient who lacks capacity in a time critical emergency, for example, the management of a head injury?

- Emergency treatment and essential clinical care should be the first priority. The senior decision-maker should use their professional judgement to determine the patient's best interests, whether planned interventions can await the recovery of capacity, and assess the amount of time it would be appropriate to spend in attempts to involve family or other relevant individuals in the decision-making process.

4) When might it be appropriate to use physical, mechanical or pharmacological restraint on a person who lacks capacity?

- If it is in their best interests to protect them from harm.

- If it is a proportionate response when compared with the potential harm faced by the person.
- If there is no less restrictive alternative.

5) A) According to the Supreme Court judgement of 19 March 2014 in the case of Cheshire West, what three elements must all be present to meet the acid test for what constitutes deprivation of liberty?

An individual is deprived of their liberty for the purposes of Article 5 of the European Convention on Human Rights if they:

- Lack the capacity to consent to their care/treatment arrangements.
- Are under continuous supervision and control.
- Are not free to leave.

B) What mechanism is in place to scrutinise the care of individuals who lack capacity to consent to restrictions that amount to a deprivation of liberty?

Amendments were made to the Mental Health Act 2007 to introduce Deprivation of Liberty Safeguards (DoLS), a framework to provide protection for the human rights of vulnerable people who lack capacity to decide about their care and treatment, where the arrangements for such care or treatment in hospitals or care homes may amount to a deprivation of their liberty, allowing scrutiny, appointment of a representative and a right to challenge.

C) What exemption to the DoLS around Article 5 may apply to patients treated in intensive care as ruled by the Court of Appeal on the 26 January 2017 in the case of Ferreira v Coroner of Inner South London (the most recent court ruling at the time of this publication — the Supreme Court refused permission to the appellant to appeal in this case in

May 2017, so the Court of Appeal judgment in Ferreira is definitive)?

The Court of Appeal ruled:

- Any deprivation of liberty resulting from the administration of life-saving treatment to a person falls outside Article 5(1) [the right to liberty]... so long as [it is] rendered unavoidable as a result of circumstances beyond the control of the authorities and is necessary to avert a real risk of serious injury or damage, and [is] kept to the minimum required for that purpose.
- The treatment must be given in good faith and is materially the same treatment as would be given to a person of sound mind with the same physical illness.
- The root cause of any loss of liberty is their physical condition, not any restrictions imposed by the hospital.

Summary of Key Points

- If a patient has capacity then they have the right to make their own decisions; no one else can consent or refuse treatment on behalf of a competent adult.
- Treatment decisions regarding patients who lack capacity should be made by the senior clinician using a collaborative approach to determine the patient's best interests, unless an attorney or deputy has been appointed.
- Restraints should only be used in a patient's best interests, proportionately and in the least restrictive way.
- The case law around the DoLS is developing so it is important to stay up to date.

References

1. Menon DK, Chatfield DA. Mental Capacity Act 2005 guidance for critical care. The Intensive Care Society, 2011. Available from: http://www.ics.ac.uk/ICS/guidelines-and-standards.aspx.

2. Crews M, Garry D, Phillips C, *et al.* Deprivation of liberty in intensive care. *J Intensive Care Soc* 2014; 15(4): 320-4.

3. Browne Jacobson LLP. ICS/FICM Guidance on MCA/DoL. The Intensive Care Society and The Faculty of Intensive Care Medicine, 2017. Available from: https://www.ficm.ac.uk/sites/default/files/updated_june_2017_-_ics_ficm_post_ferreira _briefing_note_on_mca_and_dol_final.pdf.

Malaria

1) What is malaria and can you classify its types?

Malaria

- A protozoal parasitic infection endemic in the tropics.
- Transmitted to humans via a vector — the female *Anopheles* mosquito.
- The mortality depends upon the infection type, treatment and resistance.

Types of malaria

- *Plasmodium falciparum* accounts for the largest disease burden in terms of numbers and severity, and is endemic in sub-Saharan Africa.
- *Plasmodium vivax* is the second most common and can cause severe disease. *P. vivax* predominates in the western Pacific and the Americas. There is an equal proportion of *P. falciparum* and *P. vivax* on the Indian subcontinent.
- The other types include *P. ovale*, *P. malariae* and *P. knowlesi*; each contributes a small (approximately 1%) incidence to the global disease burden but *P. knowlesi* can lead to severe disease.

2) How do patients with malaria present and what defines a severe *P. falciparum* malarial infection?

- Malaria should always be suspected when a patient has an unexplained fever.
- A travel history to a malarial endemic area within the last 30 days should be sought in all patients who have an unexplained illness.

- Further information concerning previous infections and any prophylaxis taken should also be sought.
- Classically, a swinging pyrexia is reported — this is more common with *P. vivax* and *P. ovale* than with *P. falciparum*.

Signs and symptoms include:

- Headache.
- Fatigue.
- Arthralgia and myalgia.
- Malaise.
- Anorexia.
- Diarrhoea.
- Splenomegaly.

Severe malaria is diagnosed in the presence of a parasitaemia when one or more of the following conditions is met and there is no other demonstrable cause found:

- Hypoglycaemia (blood glucose <2.2mmol/L).
- Severe anaemia (haemoglobin <70g/L with a parasite count >10,000/µL).
- Reduced conscious level (Glasgow Coma Score <11).
- Seizures (>2 in 24 hours).
- Acidosis (base excess >8mmmol/L or bicarbonate <15mmol/L).
- Renal impairment (creatinine >265µmol/L or urea >20mmol/L).
- Pulmonary oedema.
- Jaundice (bilirubin >50µmol/L.
- A coagulopathy (including clinical — spontaneous bleeding from mucous membranes).
- A parasitaemia of >10% (>500,000/µL).

N.B. for *P. vivax*, the diagnostic criteria is as above but there are no parasitaemia thresholds and for *P. knowlesi*, the parasitaemia is >100,000/μL (2%). A parasite level of over 5% is only seen with *P. falciparum*.

3) How is malaria diagnosed?

Bedside

- Temperature — serial measurements.
- Blood glucose — may be contributing to a reduced conscious level.
- Rapid diagnostic test kits — give a quick (15-20 minutes) result but offer no quantification of parasite load. They detect antigens or antibodies.
- Thromboelastography/rotational thromboelastometry (TEG®/ROTEM®) — disseminated intravascular coagulation (DIC).

Laboratory

- Thick and thin blood smears — these are more complex than they sound to prepare and interpret — usually performed three times. Thin smears on their own are less reliable. They allow for quantification of parasite load.
- Molecular testing — polymerase chain reaction (PCR) testing is useful for detecting lower-density parasitaemia.
- Full blood count — anaemia and thrombocytopenia.
- Urea and electrolytes — raised urea and creatinine.
- Liver function tests — bilirubin may be elevated.
- Clotting studies — DIC.
- Blood gases — acidosis, raised base excess, low bicarbonate.
- Blood cultures — for bacterial coinfection (*Salmonella* species have been identified as a common coinfection for *P. falciparum* malaria).
- Lumbar puncture, if unconscious, to test for bacterial meningitis.

Radiological

- Abdominal ultrasound my show splenomegaly.

4) What are the management priorities?

General measures

- An 'airway, breathing, circulation, disability and exposure' approach, especially for severe disease with organ dysfunction or low conscious level.
- Death from severe malaria can occur fast — rapid assessment and institution of anti-malarial therapy can be life-saving.
- Monitoring and supportive measures should be instituted as required:
  - IV glucose for hypoglycaemia;
  - blood transfusion for severe symptomatic anaemia;
  - oxygen for hypoxia;
  - benzodiazepines for seizures.

Medical

- If malaria prophylaxis has been taken, then the same drug should not be used for treatment.
- Paracetamol may be used for the control of fever.
- Antibiotics should be considered if bacterial coinfection is suspected or proven.
- Anti-malarials:
  - IV artesunate is the treatment of choice in adults and children (it clears parasitaemia more rapidly and demonstrates lower mortality rates than IV quinine — however, it is not licensed for use in the UK);

211

- IV quinine can be used as an alternative treatment if artesunate is not available — at a loading dose of 20mg/kg (max 1.4g) of quinine salt infused over 4 hours, then a maintenance dose of 10mg/kg every 8 hours. A 7-day course is required, but can be completed with oral therapy;
- take advice from an infectious diseases specialist — especially in cases with a very high parasite count or deterioration whilst on quinine — as artesunate may be available on a named patient basis;
- daily parasite levels should be taken to monitor treatment response.

Special

- In severe disease, consider an exchange transfusion.

5) What is the prognosis for a patient with malaria?

- Untreated *P. falciparum* infection has a mortality approaching 100%.
- The mortality for treated malaria varies depending on the setting but is still around 10% in European intensive care units and around 40% in sub-Saharan Africa.
- Pregnant women are more likely to develop severe *P. falciparum* malaria (especially in the second and third trimesters). Maternal mortality approaches 50% with premature labour and intrauterine death being common.

Summary of Key Points

- Malaria is a protozoal parasitic infection with several subtypes — the deadliest of which is *Plasmodium falciparum*.
- Consider malaria in anyone who has travelled (including stopovers) to malarial endemic areas and presents with fever.
- Blood smears are the most readily available test but require significant skill to interpret. PCR testing can be used for low parasite loads.
- IV artesunate may be better than IV quinine but is unlicensed in the UK.
- Malaria mortality remains high — prompt assessment and treatment are required.

References

1. World Health Organization. Guidelines for the treatment of malaria, 3rd ed. Geneva: WHO, 2015. Available from: http://www.who.int/malaria/publications/atoz/9789241549127/en/.

2. Dondorp AM, Fanello CI, Hendriksen IC, *et al.* Artesunate versus quinine in the treatment of severe falciparum malaria in African children (AQUAMAT): an open-label, randomised trial. *Lancet* 2010; 376: 1647.

3. Griffith KS, Lewis LS, Mali S, Parise ME. Treatment of malaria in the United States: a systematic review. *JAMA* 2007; 297: 2264.

Chronic liver failure

1) What is chronic liver failure?

Chronic liver failure is defined as a deterioration in hepatic synthetic and metabolic function, of greater than 26 weeks' duration, without encephalopathy. Acute-on-chronic liver failure refers to a patient with chronic liver disease who develops acute deterioration in liver function associated with organ dysfunction.

2) What are the systemic manifestations of chronic liver disease?

These can be classified by system:

Cardiovascular

- Coronary artery disease.
- Cardiomyopathy.
- Cardiac failure.

Respiratory

- Pulmonary hypertension.
- Pulmonary fibrosis.
- V/Q mismatching.

Neurological

- Hepatic encephalopathy.
- Polyneuropathy.
- Autonomic dysfunction.

Endocrine

- Diabetes mellitus.
- Thyroid disease.
- Hyperlipidaemia.

Haematological

- Anaemia.
- Hypersplenism.
- Neutropaenia.
- Thrombocytopenia.
- Coagulopathy.

Gastrointestinal

- Portal gastropathy and variceal disease.
- Pancreatic and biliary cancer.

Renal

- Hepatitis virus-associated nephropathy may result in mesangioproliferative, membranoproliferative or membranous glomerulonephritis.
- Hepatorenal syndrome occurs in the absence of identifiable renal disease.

Skin

- Spider naevi.
- Palmar erythema.
- Pruritis.
- Porphyria cutanea tarda.

3) How is hepatic encephalopathy graded?

The West Haven Criteria are used to grade hepatic encephalopathy from I to IV (● Table 7.1).

Table 7.1. The West Haven Criteria to grade hepatic encephalopathy.

Grade I	Behavioural change without change in level of consciousness
Grade II	Drowsiness, inappropriate behaviour, disorientation
Grade III	Marked confusion with speech that is incoherent Rousable to voice
Grade IV	Comatose; decorticate or decerebrate posturing

4) Do you know of any scoring systems used in chronic liver disease?

The Child-Pugh Score and Model of End-stage Liver Disease (MELD) Score are frequently used.

The Child-Pugh Score was originally used to prognosticate survival post-abdominal surgery. It uses the INR, albumin, bilirubin, the presence of ascites and encephalopathy to classify a patient as A, B or C (● Table 7.2). Class A gives a life expectancy of 15 to 20 years, with a predicted perioperative mortality for laparotomy of 10%. Class B gives a perioperative mortality of 30% with a life expectancy of 4 to 14 years, and Class C a perioperative mortality of 80% with a life expectancy of 1 to 2 years.

Table 7.2. The Child-Pugh Score for staging chronic liver disease.

	1 point	2 points	3 points
Bilirubin (μmol/L)	<34	34-50	>50
Albumin (g/L)	>35	28-35	<28
INR	<1/7	1.7-2.3	>2.3
Ascites	None	Mild (diuretic responsive)	Severe (unresponsive to diuresis)
Encephalopathy	None	Grade I-II	Grade III-IV

Class A: <6 points; Class B: 7-9 points; Class C: >10 points.

The MELD Score uses serum bilirubin concentration, creatinine concentration and the INR, and was initially applied to patients undergoing transjugular intrahepatic portosystemic shunt (TIPSS) procedures to predict mortality (● Table 7.3). The score was updated in 2016 to include serum sodium concentration, if the original MELD Score is >12.

MELD = 0.957 x ln(Cr) + 0.378 x ln(bilirubin) + 1.120 x ln(INR) + 0.643 (NB units in μmol/L).

A paediatric modification (PELD) Score also exists.

A score >9 is an indication for referral to a liver centre, with a score >24 used for consideration of liver transplant.

Both scoring systems may underestimate mortality in acute-on-chronic liver failure.

Table 7.3. MELD Score.

MELD Score	3-month mortality
<10	1.9%
10-19	6.0%
20-29	19.6%
30-39	52.6%
>40	71.3%

5) What may cause acute-on-chronic liver failure?

Common precipitants include infection, which may be bacterial, viral or fungal, alcoholic hepatitis, or trauma, including surgery. In around 40% of cases, no precipitating cause is found. Age, white cell count and degree of organ dysfunction are independent predictors of mortality. An exaggerated immune response is involved in the development of acute-on-chronic liver failure.

6) Outline the critical care management of acute-on-chronic liver failure.

Critical care management is supportive. Identification and treatment of the precipitating cause should be initiated. Restoration of circulating volume and maintenance of organ perfusion using vasoactive agents may be required. Cardiac output monitoring should be used to guide fluid and vasoactive agent therapy. Early administration of antibiotics when bacterial infection is suspected should be initiated. Invasive fungaemia is uncommon, although fungal colonisation is not. Albumin administration may be of benefit. Although adrenocortical failure is common, steroid administration has not been shown to improve mortality. Hepatorenal syndrome has an 85% 3-month mortality. Haemofiltration may be of use in removing circulating ammonia. A liver transplant may be used in some cases, although there is no provision for emergency liver transplantation for chronic hepatic failure in the UK.

Summary of Key Points

- Chronic liver failure has multi-systemic effects and may be graded according to the Child-Pugh Score or MELD criteria.
- Acute-on-chronic liver failure presents as acute deterioration in liver function in patients with known liver disease.
- Treatment is generally supportive, with early initiation of antimicrobial therapy if bacterial infection is suspected.
- Mortality remains high, especially if hepatorenal syndrome develops.

References

1. Arroyo V, Moreau R, Jalan R, Ginès P; EASL-CLIF Consortium CANONIC Study. Acute-on-chronic liver failure: a new syndrome that will re-classify cirrhosis. *J Hepatol* 2015; 62: S131-43.

2. Bernal W, Jalan R, Quaglia A, *et al*. Acute-on-chronic liver failure. *Lancet* 2015; 386: 1576-87.

Major haemorrhage

1) Whereabouts in the hospital might intensive care doctors become involved in caring for patients with major haemorrhage?

The areas where intensive care clinicians are likely to be involved in the management of major haemorrhage include:

- Obstetrics — where, in addition to managing the transfusion requirements, it is important to also consider drugs which increase uterine tone, bimanual compression of the uterus, packing, B-Lynch sutures and a Bakri® balloon.
- Trauma — where the haemorrhage may be compressible or non-compressible:
  - compressible — direct and indirect (tourniquet) pressure on wounds/limbs, traction to anatomical length and splinting of long bone fractures, application of a pelvic binder;
  - non-compressible — urgent surgical or interventional radiological intervention.
- Upper GI bleeds — either pre-, intra- or post-endoscopic intervention. Consider the use of terlipressin, proton pump inhibitors and a Sengstaken-Blakemore tube depending upon the aetiology of the bleeding.

In all cases of major haemorrhage, stopping the bleeding is of paramount importance. Always consider tranexamic acid, interventional radiology and the use of massive transfusion protocols to maintain adequate circulatory volume and perfusion to buy time to allow the bleeding to be controlled.

2) What are the ratios of blood products recommended for use in major haemorrhage?

Historically, this has been a contentious issue. The traditional approach to transfusion in this population was to transfuse packed red cells and then target coagulation abnormalities found on laboratory tests. This process was slow and reflected the coagulation abnormalities that were present when the tests were taken — usually around an hour prior to the result being made available.

Protocolised transfusion was established by the military during the recent conflicts in Iraq and Afghanistan with point-of-care coagulation testing improving the treatment of coagulopathy. Ratios of PRC:FFP:platelets were established at 1:1:1 during this time period.

Subsequent trials have investigated changing the ratios with the most recent showing that a ratio of 2 PRC to 1 FFP to 1 platelets showed no difference in mortality at 24 hours or 30 days but was underpowered. The same trial showed that a ratio of 1:1:1 reduced mortality from exsanguination, so the current opinion is still to transfuse blood products at a ratio of 1:1:1 guided by point-of-care testing.

3) What complications may occur as a result of massive transfusion?

These can be classified into three areas:

- Transfusion reactions:
  - haemolytic transfusion reactions — including ABO mismatched blood;
  - allergic reactions — common and usually mild, IgE-mediated;
  - bacterial infection as a result of blood product contamination;
  - transfusion-associated circulatory overload (TACO);
  - air embolism as a result of rapid infusion/pressure bags.

- Immunological complications:
  - transfusion-related acute lung injury (TRALI);
  - transfusion-associated graft vs. host disease — use irradiated products for those at risk (immunosuppressed).
- Metabolic complications:
  - hyperkalaemia — a result of haemolysis of red blood cells in storage;
  - hypocalcaemia — due to the citrate present in the transfusion products chelating calcium — this is especially apparent in patients with liver disease who cannot metabolise the citrate;
  - hypomagnesaemia — transfusion or large volumes of magnesium poor products — a dilution effect;
  - metabolic acidosis — generally from hypoperfusion as a result of the haemorrhage;
  - metabolic alkalosis — metabolised citrate produces bicarbonate so this may cause a metabolic alkalosis especially in the presence of renal dysfunction;
  - hypothermia — rapid transfusion of blood products if not heated to body temperature; usually patient exposure for assessment and intervention contributes significantly to heat loss.

4) What are the endpoint targets in massive transfusion?

The target in massive transfusion is to support end-organ perfusion, oxygen delivery and coagulation, and minimise metabolic compromise whilst interventions occur to stop the bleeding. Whilst this is being achieved, and major haemorrhage is ongoing, the following endpoints should be aimed for:

- Temperature >36°C.
- pH >7.2.
- Lactate <2mmol/L.
- Base excess >-6.

- Haemoglobin >100g/L during bleeding; >80g/L is acceptable once controlled.
- Fibrinogen >1.5g/L.
- Platelets >100 x10^9/L.
- Ionised calcium >1mmol/L.
- Potassium <5.5mmol/L.
- Normal coagulation guided by point-of-care testing.
- A mean arterial pressure of >65mmHg (may initially permit hypotensive resuscitation to limit haemorrhage prior to surgical/ interventional radiological control).

5) Is there a role for whole blood transfusion in major haemorrhage?

Up until the 1970s, whole blood transfusion was the norm and remains so to this day in much of the world. The switch to component therapy by the developed world occurred without much evidence to suggest it was superior and indeed the subsequent 40 years of practice has brought us back to using component products in ratios which mimic whole blood.

However, there may be problems with whole blood:

- Stored whole blood loses platelet function within approximately 48 hours.
- Fresh warm whole blood has logistical difficulties and increases the risk of transmission of infections.

There have been several studies which have demonstrated increased survival with the use of fresh warm whole blood compared to blood component therapy. Therefore, there is likely to be a role for fresh warm whole blood in certain circumstances and populations, but it is unlikely to be reintroduced into routine practice for major haemorrhage.

Summary of Key Points

- Massive transfusion can occur anywhere in the hospital but most commonly as a result of obstetric haemorrhage, trauma or upper GI bleeding.
- All major haemorrhage patients should receive tranexamic acid and be considered for interventional radiology.
- Transfusion ratios of 1:1:1 PRC:FFP:platelets are currently recommended.
- Massive transfusion is not without its complications and metabolic derangement needs careful management.
- There may be a role for fresh warm whole blood, but it is not yet defined.

References

1. HA Doughty, T Woolley, GOR Thomas. Massive transfusion. *J R Army Med Corps* 2011; 157(3 Suppl 1): S277-83.

2. Holcomb JB, Tilley BC, Baraniuk S, *et al*; PROPPR Study Group. Transfusion of plasma, platelets, and red blood cells in a 1:1:1 vs a 1:1:2 ratio and mortality in patients with severe trauma: the PROPPR randomized clinical trial.. *JAMA* 2015; 313(5): 471-82.

3. Davies RL Should whole blood replace the shock pack? *J R Army Med Corps* 2016; 162(1): 5-7.

4. Spinella PC, Perkins JG, Grathwohl KW, *et al*. Warm fresh whole blood is independently associated with improved survival for patients with combat-related traumatic injuries. *J Trauma* 2009; 66(Suppl 4): S69-76.

Thrombotic thrombocytopenic purpura (TTP)

1) What is TTP and how can it be subclassified?

TTP is a thrombotic microangiopathy caused by reduced activity in the enzyme that breaks down von Willebrand factor, therefore leading to over-activation of platelet aggregation and clot formation in capillaries. The excessive consumption of platelets leads to thrombocytopenia.

There are two underlying causes for TTP:

- Autoimmune TTP — a condition with an incidence of approximately three cases per million per year. An antibody is formed against the von Willebrand factor cleaving protease (ADAMTS13). It occurs more commonly in women.
- Hereditary TTP — an autosomal recessive condition where mutations in the ADAMTS13 gene occur (several different mutations are described) leading to a deficiency in the von Willebrand factor cleaving protease.

2) What are the clinical manifestations of autoimmune TTP and how does TTP lead to death?

Autoimmune TTP manifests itself as a severe microangiopathic haemolytic anaemia (MAHA) and usually presents in young adults. It can be associated with other autoimmune diseases such as systemic lupus erythematosus, and with pregnancy. Symptoms of MAHA include:

- Fatigue.
- Petechial haemorrhages — especially as a result of minor trauma.
- Dyspnoea — multiple small pulmonary emboli causing shunt, possibly causing some effect on the right side of the heart.
- Bleeding from other sites — particularly the gastrointestinal tract.

227

- Chronic low-grade fever.
- Fluctuating neurological symptoms — akin to transient ischaemic attacks but may be central or peripheral in their aetiology.

Patients may present with relatively minor symptoms and the diagnosis may not be made until after investigations have been carried out or they may present critically unwell with ischaemic symptoms.

The primary cause of death is myocardial ischaemia caused by platelet-rich thrombi in the coronary arteries. Mortality before effective treatment became available approached 90%.

3) What investigations should you request if you suspect TTP?

Most of the investigations for TTP are laboratory-based and include:

- Full blood count — to assess platelet level (although not platelet function) and anaemia — secondary to haemolysis as a result of the microangiopathic emboli.
- Blood film — will likely be automatically triggered by the presence of thrombocytopenia on the full blood count and will show haemolysis and platelet aggregation.
- Coagulation studies — may be normal or in severe cases may show disseminated intravascular coagulation (DIC), again as a result of the microangiopathic emboli.
- Urea and electrolytes — may show elevated creatinine in acute renal failure secondary to ischaemia from emboli to the kidney.
- Serum lactate dehydrogenase, bilirubin and reticulocyte count — indicative of the haemolytic component of the condition.
- Stool and blood cultures may be useful in consideration of the differential diagnosis, as may HIV and hepatitis serology (see below).
- Direct antiglobulin test (DAT/Coombs test) — will be negative in TTP.

- Testing of ADAMTS13 activity and inhibition — ideally the sample should be sent before treatment is instigated. Activity of <10% is diagnostic. Not all laboratories will be able to process this test, so the result may not be immediately available. Treatment should not be delayed waiting for this confirmatory test.
- Genetic testing is available for the mutations which occur in hereditary TTP and should be considered for family members of the affected person if positive.

Other investigations include:

- CT or MRI of the brain and/or spinal cord if neurological symptoms predominate.

4) What are the treatment options available for TTP?

- The mainstay of treatment for TTP is plasma exchange and this should be instigated as soon as possible and thereafter continued daily until 2 days after complete remission occurs (normal platelet count). Plasma exchange not only removes the autoantibodies responsible for autoimmune TTP, but replaces the von Willebrand factor cleaving protease with donor enzymes, and is therefore thought to be superior to plasmapheresis which would only remove the antibodies and not replace the enzymes.
- The addition of steroids is recommended by most haematologists despite the lack of randomised controlled trials proving their efficacy. They are assumed to dampen the autoimmune process and reduce the production of autoantibody. Observational studies suggest that they reduce the number of cycles of plasma exchange required.
- Other immunosuppressive agents are not routinely used but rituximab is indicated for use in severe or relapsing disease.

5) What other conditions present in a similar way to TTP?

The differential diagnosis of TTP includes all other conditions which present with MAHA, incorporating:

- Drug-induced thrombotic microangiopathy (TMA) — similar to TTP but without the ADAMTS13 involvement. It occurs as a result of administration of drugs including quinine and quetiapine. The mechanism is thought to be an interaction of the drug with the walls of arterioles causing microthrombi formation.
- Shigella toxin-mediated haemolytic uraemic syndrome (HUS) — causes a TMA as a result of a diarrhoeal illness (hence the need for stool and blood cultures to be taken as part of the investigative process), with acute renal failure a feature.
- Complement-mediated TMA — can be hereditary or acquired.

Summary of Key Points

- Autoimmune TTP is a rare but potentially fatal condition predominantly affecting young women.
- Clinical manifestations may be mild or severe and are as a result of microthrombosis.
- Death occurs due to thrombosis in the coronary arteries.
- The main treatment is plasma exchange which should be instigated immediately.
- There are many other TMA syndromes and considerable overlap with haemolytic uraemic syndrome.

References

1. Fujimura Y, Matsumoto M, Isonishi A, *et al*. Natural history of Upshaw-Schulman syndrome based on ADAMTS13 gene analysis in Japan. *J Thromb Haemost* 2011; 9 Suppl 1: 283.

2. George JN, Nester CM. Syndromes of thrombotic microangiopathy. *N Engl J Med* 2014; 371: 654.

3. Amorosi EL, Ultmann JE. Thrombotic thrombocytopenic purpura: report of 16 cases and review of the literature. *Medicine* (Baltimore) 1966; 45: 139.

4. Blombery P, Scully M. Management of thrombotic thrombocytopenic purpura: current perspectives. *J Blood Med* 2014; 5: 15.

5. Lim W, Vesely SK, George JN. The role of rituximab in the management of patients with acquired thrombotic thrombocytopenic purpura. *Blood* 2015; 125: 1526.

Neuroleptic malignant syndrome

1) What is neuroleptic malignant syndrome?

Neuroleptic malignant syndrome

- Neuroleptic malignant syndrome (NMS) is a rare but life-threatening complication of neuroleptic (antipsychotic) medication administration.
- NMS usually occurs within 2 weeks after initiation of neuroleptic treatment, or shortly after a dose increase.
- It is characterised by hyperthermia (temperature >38°C), muscle rigidity, altered mental status and autonomic dysfunction.
- It has a mortality rate of 10-20%.

2) Which neuroleptic agents are implicated?

- NMS is more commonly associated with the typical higher-potency neuroleptic agents such as haloperidol and fluphenazine.
- It can also be associated with lower-potency agents such as chlorpromazine, but can be associated with any antipsychotic medication including atypical agents such as clozapine, risperidone and olanzapine.

3) A) Briefly outline the pathophysiology of NMS.

- Dopamine receptor antagonism is thought to be the cause of NMS.
- D2 receptor blockade in the hypothalamus, nigrostriatal pathways and spinal cord results in temperature dysregulation, muscle rigidity and tremor.
- Neuroleptics can cause an exaggerated calcium release in the sarcoplasmic reticulum of skeletal muscle resulting in increased

contractility also contributing to hyperthermia, rigidity and muscle necrosis.

B) What further complications may characterise NMS?

● The intense hypermetabolic reaction that occurs in skeletal muscle leads to severe muscle rigidity, extensive rhabdomyolysis, hyperkalaemia and renal failure (mortality rises to 50% with renal failure).

C) What features constitute a diagnosis of NMS and what are the differential diagnoses?

● A diagnosis of NMS requires hyperthermia, muscle rigidity and other features of NMS including:
  - change in mental status;
  - autonomic instability (labile blood pressure, tachycardia, diaphoresis, incontinence);
  - tremor;
  - leucocytosis;
  - laboratory evidence of muscle injury (raised CK, myoglobinuria);
  - metabolic acidosis;
  - psychomotor agitation and delirium;
  - tachypnoea;
  - hypoxaemia.
● Other neuroleptic-induced reactions include:
  - acute dystonia;
  - acute akathisia;
  - tardive dyskinesia;
  - parkinsonism.
● Other differential diagnoses include:
  - lethal catatonia;
  - serotonin syndrome;
  - malignant hyperthermia;

- CNS infections and other sepsis;
- acute intermittent porphyria;
- tetanus;
- thyroid storm;
- heat stroke;
- amphetamine/anticholinergic/cocaine/lithium/MAOI/SSRI toxicity;
- phaeochromocytoma.

4) What investigations would you order for someone suspected of having NMS?

Bedside

- Urine dipstick and analysis — myoglobinuria.
- ABG — metabolic acidosis.

Laboratory

- Full blood count — leucocytosis, thrombocytosis.
- Renal biochemistry — dehydration, hyperkalaemia, hyperphosphataemia, hypocalcaemia, renal failure.
- CK, LDH, uric acid, myoglobin — elevated in rhabdomyolysis.
- Liver function tests — elevated AST, ALT.
- Coagulation profile — in thromboembolic disorders or DIC.
- Toxicology — to exclude overdose.

Radiological

- CT and/or MRI brain — to rule out other conditions causing altered mental status.
- CXR — for suspected aspiration pneumonia.

Other

- Septic screen — including lumbar puncture (post-CT brain excluding structural lesions) to exclude other causes of fever and altered mental status.

5) What are the management priorities for NMS?

General supportive measures

- Resuscitation to follow an 'airway, breathing, circulation, disability and exposure' approach.
- Withdrawal of the causative agent.
- Reversal of hyperthermia; common methods include:
  - cooling blankets;
  - cooled IV fluids;
  - ice packs;
  - endovascular cooling with a heat-exchange catheter, e.g. Thermogard XP®;
  - extracorporeal circuit cooling.
- Renal replacement therapy — to clear hyperkalaemia and plasma toxins released in rhabdomyolysis (also a method of extracorporeal cooling).

Pharmacological

- Dantrolene — muscle relaxation, dosing: IV bolus 2.5mg/kg, followed by 1mg/kg boluses as required every 5-10 minutes to a maximum of 10mg/kg.
- Dopaminergic drugs, e.g. bromocriptine and amantadine — antagonise the effect of neuroleptic drugs at dopaminergic receptors.
- Antipyretics, e.g. paracetamol.

Summary of Key Points

- Neuroleptic malignant syndrome (NMS) is a rare complication of antipsychotic medication administration with a mortality rate of 10-20%.
- It is characterised by hyperthermia, muscle rigidity, altered mental status and autonomic dysfunction, and may proceed to rhabdomyolysis and renal failure.
- Dopamine receptor antagonism is the likely underlying cause of NMS.
- NMS requires rapid admission to intensive care, withdrawal of the causative agent, temperature correction, other supportive measures, dantrolene and bromocriptine.

References

1.   Mathieu S, Hutchings S, Craig G. Neuroleptic malignant syndrome: severe hyperthermia treated with endovascular cooling. *J Intensive Care Soc* 2010; 11(3): 187-9.

2.   Benzer T, Mancini MC, Shamovitz GZ. Neuroleptic malignant syndrome. Medscape 2016. Available from: http://emedicine.medscape.com/article/816018.

Intensive care scoring systems

1) What is the purpose of scoring systems?

There are three main purposes of scoring systems in healthcare:

- To assess the severity of a condition for individual patients, e.g. the Glasgow Coma Score allows us to quantify the level of consciousness and is validated against outcome with regard to traumatic head injury. This type of score also allows the communication of severity between health professionals who should have similar knowledge about what a certain score means, and allows treatments to be targeted to appropriate patients.
- To predict survival, morbidity or mortality in a certain population, e.g. the Acute Physiology and Chronic Health Evaluation (APACHE) score allows us to retrospectively look at outcomes and compare them to the severity scoring of patients admitted to intensive care.

N.B. there is significant crossover within the above two purposes — severity scoring for individual patients may be used to allow comparison of patient population outcomes with similar severity scores.

- For audit and research, to allow comparison of performance across similar areas of healthcare provision, e.g. in the UK, the Intensive Care National Audit and Research Centre (ICNARC) receives data submitted from all intensive care units. It then analyses this data and places each intensive care unit on a funnel plot with similar units by size and population to allow comparison.

2) How can you classify scoring systems?

Scoring systems can be classified into:

- Disease- or organ-specific — for example, the Child Pugh and MELD scores in liver disease.
- Anatomical scores — such as the Injury Severity Score (ISS) which takes nine anatomical areas and scores them between 1-6, depending upon the extent of injury in each area. The worst three scores are taken, squared and then added together with the score ranging from 1-75 (maximum score is 75 being $5^2+5^2+5^2$; any score of 6 in any body region automatically achieves a score of 75).
- Intervention scoring — for example, the Therapeutic Intervention Scoring System (TISS), whereby the more interventions a patient requires the higher their score and the sicker they are perceived to be.
- Physiological scores — such as APACHE, the Simplified Acute Physiology Score (SAPS), the Multiple Organ Dysfunction Score (MODS) and the Physiological and Operative Severity Score for the enUmeration of Mortality (P-POSSUM), which take physiological variables with the premise that the more deranged these are the sicker a cohort of patients is and the worse the outcome.
- Ongoing assessment scores — these take data over a longer period of time rather than at a single point to allow assessment of response to therapy, for example, the Sequential Organ Failure Assessment (SOFA) score and the National Early Warning Score (NEWS).

3) Tell me about the APACHE II scoring system.

The APACHE II score was developed during the 1980s and is calculated on the basis of the patient's age, their background health including recent surgery, chronic organ insufficiency and immunocompromised state. This is collected along with the worst derangement of 12 physiological variables measured in the first 24 hours of acute illness including:

- Temperature.
- Mean arterial pressure.
- PaO_2.
- Heart rate.
- Respiratory rate.
- GCS.
- White cell count.
- Haematocrit.
- Serum sodium.
- Serum potassium.
- Creatinine.
- Arterial pH.

Each variable is weighted from 0-4 with more weight given to further deviation from normal values:

- The maximum score is 71.
- A score of 25 represents a predicted mortality of 50%.
- A score of 35 represents a predicted mortality of 80%.

It is the most common scoring system used in intensive care worldwide despite the fact that it has been superseded by APACHE III and IV — both of which have copyrighted algorithms so the cost to upgrade to these has been a significant factor in the adoption.

4) What are the potential problems with scoring systems?

Scoring systems are an important part of intensive care audit and research but they are not without their problems including:

- Validity — the populations in which they were developed may be significantly different from those to which we are applying the scores and this may invalidate the outcome measures, e.g. most scoring systems are only valid for use within the first 24 hours of intensive care admission and therefore their repeated use past this time may not give the outcome expected.
- Bias — both within the scoring system itself and as a result of the data input level.
- Comparison — especially between different intensive care units — no two units are completely identical and using scoring systems to say that one is better or worse than another is a potentially hazardous thing to do in the current climate of healthcare reform.
- Scoring systems are almost universally population-based and therefore cannot be reliably applied to the individual patient presented in front of the clinician.

5)   What would an ideal ICU scoring system look like?

An ideal ICU scoring system would have the following qualities:

- Simple — using routinely available patient information and results.
- Objective (not subjective).
- Validated in all patient populations with a high sensitivity and specificity.
- Able to be used in countries all over the world.
- Predict outcome for both the individual patient and on a population basis.
- Independent of patient variables.
- Allow a high level of discrimination between patients.
- Be free to use and easily available.
- Not affected by user bias.
- Be linear in scale — doubling the score would double the likelihood of an adverse outcome and make the score easier to understand.

Summary of Key Points

- Scoring systems can be useful for individual patients or more commonly for population prediction.
- They can be classified by the way that they measure variables.
- The most common ICU scoring system is APACHE II.
- Scoring systems are not without their problems which may be so significant that it renders them invalid in certain circumstances/ populations.
- An ideal scoring system would address the shortcomings of the systems currently in use.

References

1. Knaus WA, Draper EA, Wagner DP, Zimmerman JE. APACHE II: a severity of disease classification system. *Crit Care Med* 1985; 13(10): 818-29.

Alcohol poisoning (ethanol and methanol)

1) Classify the stages of ethanol poisoning.

Ethanol is the alcohol found in widely available 'alcoholic' beverages. The ethanol contained within them is rapidly absorbed from the gastrointestinal tract. It is metabolised at a constant rate which may increase in people who are regular and 'tolerant' drinkers.

These escalating ethanol blood levels cause the following sequelae:

- 200-500mg/L causes disinhibition, excitation and emotional ability.
- 500-1000mg/L leads to decreased reaction time and judgement with a loss of fine motor skills.
- 1000-2000mg/L may start to obtund consciousness with autonomic dysfunction.
- 2000-4500mg/L causes depressed conscious level and may cause hypoglycaemia and precipitate seizures.
- >4500mg/L causes loss of consciousness and protective airway reflexes, respiratory depression, hypoglycaemia, seizures and may be lethal.

In general, the fatal dose is 5-8g/kg body weight (3g/kg in children).

2) How does methanol toxicity differ from ethanol toxicity?

Ethanol

- The precise mechanism of central nervous system (CNS) effects is unknown.

- Ethanol is a secondary alcohol and undergoes some metabolism to ketones.
- Ethanol is also metabolised to acetone which is formed more rapidly than it can be eliminated in significant ethanol ingestion. The acetone levels increase and have a direct and synergistic CNS depressant effect in addition to the unmetabolised ethanol.
- Ethanol is significantly less toxic than methanol or ethylene glycol.

Methanol

- Is a primary and 'toxic' alcohol.
- It is metabolised by oxidation to formic acid (via alcohol dehydrogenase and aldehyde dehydrogenase).
- Formic acid is a toxic substance which causes severe metabolic acidosis, blindness, renal failure and may be lethal.
- Methanol toxicity will initially cause an elevated osmolar gap which then falls in conjunction with a rise in the anion gap as formic acid is produced.

3) How are osmolar and anion gaps calculated?

Osmolar gap

- The difference between the measured osmolality and the calculated osmolarity.
- Osmolarity is calculated: $2(Na^+ + K^+) + $ glucose $ + $ urea.
- The normal osmolar gap is <10 (no units as it is a pragmatic clinical aid using different units: osmolality = mOsm/kg and osmolarity = mOsm/L).

- A high osmolar gap suggests the presence of significant amounts of an abnormal solute, e.g.:
  - methanol;
  - ethanol — if the blood ethanol level is measured, then this can be added into the calculated osmolarity to ensure that there is not another underlying solute contributing to the high osmolar gap;
  - ethylene glycol;
  - mannitol;
  - propylene glycol — the solvent used to deliver intravenous lorazepam and diazepam, so this may cause iatrogenic elevation of the osmolar gap.

Anion gap

- Useful in metabolic acidosis to determine the presence of unmeasured anions.
- Calculated by: $Na^+ - (Cl^- + HCO_3^-)$.
- The normal value for the anion gap depends upon the patient's albumin and phosphate levels but is typically between 4-12mmol/L.
- High anion gap metabolic acidosis is due to the presence of organic acids, e.g.:
  - ketones;
  - lactate;
  - urea;
  - toxic acids — formic acid, ethylene glycol, methanol;
  - drugs — paracetamol, salicylates, isoniazid, metformin, etc.
- Normal anion gap metabolic acidosis is due to bicarbonate loss secondary to:
  - renal tubular acidosis;
  - gastrointestinal losses, i.e. diarrhoea and vomiting, or high-output stoma losses;
  - diuretic use — acetazolamide;
  - excess chloride administration.

4) What antidotes are available for methanol poisoning?

The mainstay of treatment for methanol poisoning is to block the pathway of metabolism to toxic metabolites:

- Ethanol — has a greater affinity for alcohol dehydrogenase than methanol so will prevent the breakdown of methanol (which will then be slowly excreted [half-life of 30-50 hours]). Problems with the use of ethanol as an antidote include:
    - raising the osmolar gap making it more difficult to monitor the response to treatment;
    - it is difficult to maintain the ethanol concentration at the appropriate level and the patient may require ongoing sedation to mitigate the euphoric effects of a high plasma ethanol level.
- Fomepizole — a preferred antidote for the following reasons:
    - plasma concentrations do not need to be monitored;
    - it can be used safely in patients with liver failure, those taking metronidazole or those who are pregnant;
    - it can be given as a dose every 12 hours rather than as a continuous infusion.

It is important to note that fomepizole is expensive — in the UK it costs approximately £5000 for a treatment course following methanol toxicity.

5) What are the general management priorities for methanol poisoning?

General

- Ensure airway patency and secure if necessary.
- There is NO role for activated charcoal but there may be a role for nasogastric tube insertion and drainage of stomach contents to prevent further absorption.

- Measure blood glucose and correct as required — likely to be hypoglycaemic.
- Obtain a 12-lead ECG — specific abnormalities include a prolonged QT and broad QRS complexes in severe acidosis.
- Send blood samples for U&Es, including chloride and bicarbonate, liver function tests, measured osmolality, and arterial blood gases. N.B. the lactate on blood gas machines may measure formic acid as lactate so may be artificially high compared with the laboratory lactate value. Measure methanol and ethanol levels.
- Give IV vitamin B complex if there is a history of alcohol abuse.

Medical

- Use ethanol or fomepizole antidotes as available.
- Give folinic acid at a dose of 1-2mg/kg QDS or folic acid 50mg QDS, as this enhances the breakdown of any formic acid which may have already formed.
- Rehydrate with IV fluids.
- If metabolic acidosis persists consider the use of intravenous bicarbonate.

Special

- Haemodialysis (and to a lesser extent haemofiltration) should be considered in severe toxicity to remove methanol, formic acid and formaldehyde. Haemodialysis reduces the effective half-life of methanol to 4 hours (from 30-50 hours with antidote use alone [8 hours with haemofiltration]).

The endpoint of haemodialysis or antidote treatment is an undetectable plasma methanol level.

Summary of Key Points

- Ethanol is a very common drug of abuse which is potentially fatal at high concentrations.
- Ethanol is directly toxic and synergistic with acetone (its metabolite), whereas methanol is in itself non-toxic but its metabolite is extremely toxic.
- Osmolar and anion gaps can be useful in recognising the causes of a metabolic acidosis.
- Fomepizole is a superior antidote for methanol poisoning than ethanol but is more expensive.
- Supportive measures and antidotes are the mainstay of treatment, but consider the use of haemodialysis in severe toxicity.

References

1. Gennari FJ. Current concepts. Serum osmolality. Uses and limitations. *N Engl J Med* 1984; 310(2): 102-5.
2. Kraut JA, Madias NE. Serum anion gap: its uses and limitations in clinical medicine. *Clin J Am Soc Nephrol* 2007; 2(1): 162-74.
3. Brent J, Mcmartin K, Philips S, *et al.* Fomepizole in the treatment of methanol poisoning. *N Engl J Med* 2001; 344: 24-2.

Index